special praise for

•••••••••••••••••••••

my life as a
border collie

"Nancy Johnston's advice for codependents a͟ ͟ ͟ose who love them
finds a new voice in *My Life as a Border Collie*. Johnston draws on life with
her own border collie, Daisy, to give the reader a whole new way of
thinking about codependency, as she taps Daisy's behaviors to illustrate
both the good and the less-optimal sides of loyalty, devotion, service,
and other attributes. The range of those behaviors, from successful to
exasperating to self-defeating—and back, thank goodness—has never
been clearer than in this wise and witty book. Sit! Stay! READ!"

Lisa Tracy
Journalist and Author of *Objects of Our Affection:*
Uncovering My Family's Past, One Chair, Pistol, and Pickle Fork at a Time

"Using her border collie, Daisy, and the characteristics of border
collies as a background, Johnston has found an unprecedented and
extremely clever way to teach readers about codependence. Her
training as a licensed professional counselor and licensed substance
abuse treatment practitioner clearly helps Johnston elucidate this
important topic, but what shines through is her personal experience
with codependence, her love and tremendous respect for her dog,
Daisy, and her intense admiration for this remarkable breed called the
border collie."

Mary R. Burch, PhD
Board Certified Behavior Analyst (BCBA-D) and Author of
The Border Collie: An Owner's Guide to a Happy Healthy Pet

"*My Life as a Border Collie* is an informative and entertaining book that examines the syndrome of codependency as expressed in the life and tales of the author's border collie. To the attentive observer, 'man's best friend' teaches living lessons about the paradoxes of human nature. I will return to this book over and over again as I seek freedom from my learned, self-defeating thinking and behaviors. This book is a highly valuable addition to the personal library of anyone working on recovery from codependency."

David L. Nelson, MD

"Nancy Johnston has brought a balanced approach to the subject of out-of-balance relationships. She begins with a clinical and academic look, which she then brings to life by using both her own experiences and those of her beloved border collie, Daisy.

"I love the way the book is formatted, with a near perfect balance of vulnerability and self-disclosure, stories of Nancy's own life, and her equally charming dog, Daisy in 'Tales Told'; practical skills in 'Lessons Learned'; and academic information in 'The Codependency Story.'

"I appreciate her diligent review of what is new in the field and the way she ties it together in such an informative, yet utterly charming manner! Nancy has moved to the forefront in the field of codependence."

Margaret Cress, LMFT
Cofacilitator of Codependence Camp

"I have read multiple self-help books about codependency through the years. Nancy's book, however, provided the best visualization for recognizing codependent behavior via her continuum. For the first time I can keep an awareness of whether my behavior reflects 'you've gone too far'

special praise for
••••••••••••••••••••
*my life as a
border collie*

or if I was responding in the 'this is okay' end. The continuum has quickly become a supportive self-awareness mind exercise for me.

"Nancy Johnston presents a refreshing method of recognizing our true feelings in response to various situations in a positive manner."

Lauren K. Keating, DVM

"In *My Life as a Border Collie*, Nancy Johnston has created an endearing, entertaining, and highly practical prescription for those of us who want to recover our 'selves.' The comparison of her thoughts and behaviors to that of her sweet canine companion, Daisy, is truly unique and fascinating. I started the book with interest and couldn't put it down. I love this book!"

Hope Hennessey
Editor and Life Coach

"A clinically relevant and useful book. Nancy Johnston provides a continuum of behaviors from which readers can self-identify as healthy or less healthy. She illustrates the consequences of these behaviors through stories about her own life and through case studies from her practice. She then provides specific actions for self-directed change for any reader motivated to embrace health.

"I learned quite a bit about border collies too!"

Molly O'Dell, MD

"*My Life as a Border Collie* is a remarkable, energetic, and joyful book ... containing many great lessons for all of us whether we are dog owners or not. Its lessons range far beyond her 'life as a border collie,' to include how to be in a family, how to approach the world sanely in an insane age, and how to really love. I recommend it highly!"

Katie Letcher Lyle
Author

"Nancy's insights make a wealth of research easily accessible to those of us trying to navigate life with more self-awareness—building on the good aspects of our border collieness while maintaining a thoughtful balance that makes life the richer."

Phyllis R. Parker
Writer and Teacher

"*My Life as a Border Collie* made the dog lover, the therapist, and the recovering codependent in me smile with appreciation. Nancy cleverly weaves in an overview of the best literature on codependency and recovery as she sheds the light of everyday life on it with stories of herself and her dog Daisy and their similarities. Using a border collie as her mirror to her own strengths and struggles, she explores many stumbling blocks to recovery in a lighthearted manner. Bravo, Nancy, for providing a template for recovering readers to look at themselves honestly without taking themselves too seriously. I know I have 'dog-eared' several sections to revisit."

Lois B. Horne, EdS, LPC, LSATP

my life
as a
border collie

my life
as a
border collie

FREEDOM FROM CODEPENDENCY

NANCY L. JOHNSTON, MS, LPC, LSATP

CENTRAL RECOVERY PRESS

Central Recovery Press

Central Recovery Press (CRP) is committed to publishing exceptional materials addressing addiction treatment, recovery, and behavioral healthcare topics, including original and quality books, audio/visual communications, and web-based new media. Through a diverse selection of titles, we seek to contribute a broad range of unique resources for professionals, recovering individuals and their families, and the general public.

For more information, visit www.centralrecoverypress.com.

Central Recovery Press, Las Vegas, NV 89129

© 2012 by Nancy L. Johnston
All rights reserved. Published 2012.
Printed in the United States of America.

No part of this publication may be reproduced, stored in a retrieval system, or transmitted in any form or by any means, electronic, mechanical, photocopying, recording, or otherwise, without the written permission of the publisher.

Publisher: Central Recovery Press
3321 N. Buffalo Drive
Las Vegas, NV 89129

17 16 15 14 13 12   1 2 3 4 5

ISBN-13: 978-1-936290-92-5 (paper)
ISBN-13: 978-1-937612-00-9 (e-book)

Author photo by Monty Johnston. Used with permission.

Publisher's Note: Central Recovery Press books represent the experiences and opinions of their authors only. Every effort has been made to ensure that events, institutions, and statistics presented in our books as facts are accurate and up-to-date. To protect their privacy, the names of some of the people and institutions in this book have been changed.

Cover design and interior layout by Heather Kern, Popshop Studio Design

beginnings
How This All Came to Be

tales and lessons

never-endings

*M*y *Life as a Border Collie: Freedom from Codependency* is not a direct sequel to *Disentangle: When You've Lost Your Self in Someone Else*, but it does build on the foundational concepts and tools offered in *Disentangle* as a means of finding and strengthening our self.

The overall concept for *My Life as a Border Collie* came to me ten years ago as a result of both my recovery from codependency and my relationship with Daisy, our border collie. Over these ten years, I have published, presented, and taught the material in *Disentangle,* and thus expanded my own understanding of its contents and my ability to convey my understanding to others. *My Life as a Border Collie* has benefited from these developments of the *Disentangle* material. And while *My Life as a Border Collie* makes references to the codependency recovery ideas in *Disentangle,* it goes well beyond *Disentangle* in its own unique and rich way, extending our understanding of codependency as well as ways to manage our selves so that our very strengths do not become our weaknesses.

In the Preface to *Disentangle* I wrote the following, which still applies here:

> *As you may have already noticed in my writing here, I am separating the word "self" from possessives such as "my" and "your." This is intentional on my part. I want to emphasize the word "self." It is, in fact, what this book is largely about, and I am interested in helping the reader to keep that word, that concept, that important reality in mind. Disentangle is about finding our self when we have lost it in someone else. It is about learning how to connect with our self and then knowing how to respond to it in ways that make us stronger, clearer, and more serene.*

My Life as a Border Collie is also about our self-development. It is about learning to focus on our self in healthy, informed, and empowering ways that enable us to have peace within our self and within our relationships. It is about learning how to notice and intervene on our own behalf when we are about to let a positive characteristic of our self become a problem. Many tales and lessons from Daisy and me await you within these pages that provide information and inspiration to help you in this work on behalf of your self.

I am pleased to offer you more of what I continue to learn about codependency and about my self.

I hope this may be useful for your self as well.

Nancy L. Johnston
May, 2012

acknowledgments
....

To my family members, friends, colleagues, and clients,
who have been anywhere from curious to serious
about codependency and its relevance
to a healthy self and healthy relationships.

To Central Recovery Press
for their deep understanding and support
of this important topic.

And to Daisy for many years of
loving and learning.

I thank you all.

beginnings

· ·

how this all came to be

*W*ithout being trained to know basic good manners and how to engage in activities that can stimulate the active border collie mind while still being acceptable to the minds of their human friends, border collies can become absolute maniacs.[1]

—Mary Burch
author of *The Border Collie:
An Owner's Guide to a Happy Healthy Pet*

W hen John, our flat-coat retriever mix, was fourteen years old, we had to euthanize him. It was a horribly sad day for my husband Monty and me, even though we knew without any doubt that we needed to help him pass on. For a couple of years prior to his death, he had seizures intermittently. They had become more frequent and damaging to his body. We came to understand they were likely caused by a brain tumor. He had been a wonderful dog, friend, and companion. My husband had named him John, because he had no sons and wanted to use this name. John was a son of ours.

On the day of his passing, John lay on the floor of the veterinarian's examining room, seemingly comfortable but with very little life in him. After hours of walking, talking, and crying, we made our final decision and let our dear John go.

As life would have it, we had to leave town later that day to attend the wedding of a good friend. As we left, through my tears, I said to Monty, "Maybe when we come back there will be a dog on our front porch with a little note that says, 'John sent me.'"

That was October 1996.

When we returned home several days later, there was no dog or note. That was okay. In fact, that was good. Necessary grief takes necessary time. Neither of us really wanted to fill our holes of loss too soon with another dog. Grief needed to take its natural course.

And so it did.

In December 1996, Monty, our eight-year-old daughter Grace, and I drove out of our country driveway one night, heading up the hill from our house to the elementary school to see Grace in the Christmas program. There, at the end of our eighth-of-a-mile driveway, were three dogs, looking lost. They stood practically still in our headlights. We decided it was likely a mother dog and two of her somewhat grown-up pups. We felt sad for them, believing they had likely been abandoned, deserted by their owner.

Sad, yes, but we drove away, up the hill for our brief ride to the school. As we returned home an hour and a half later, there were the dogs again in our headlights as we made a switchback turn. Again, "oohs" and "ahhs" of sympathy and sadness for the dogs, but on we went to home.

I did not even think of them again that night, though our backyard light could well have illuminated a path for them straight to our back door.

The next morning I was getting Grace ready for school, and it was then that I thought of the dogs again. I wondered what had happened to them during the night and decided to do a quick look for them after I left Grace at school. I did not mention this to her.

So back out the driveway we went, winding up the hill to her school—no dogs in sight.

I hugged and kissed Grace good-bye and headed home.

Where might they be?

Maybe at the dumpsters a half mile away? They were not there.

Maybe wandering the neighborhood? They were not to be seen.

I was giving up on this brief, random excursion as I headed back down the hill to our river house when, just as I came over the ridge of a hill, there was one of the dogs, standing off to the side of the road. I was able to pull off and stop.

I turned off my car and slowly got out. I walked around to the back of the car and squatted down to speak to the dog, which had not moved. As I opened my arms and hands to her, she was willing to come to me and allow me to pick her up. She must have been around twenty-five pounds, black with white markings on her paws, chest, and face. She did not resist me at all.

I found her on land just above our property, practically in our yard. I did not want to scare her by putting her in my car, so I carried her down the path to our backyard.

My husband was still asleep in bed. I was able to carry the dog to just outside the window where he was sleeping. I called to him to wake up and look, and I said, "Here is the dog John sent."

It appeared that the dog had spent the night sleeping on the land just above us, waiting for the morning and her new people to find her. The other dogs were gone, and I never saw them again.

Daisy has now lived with us for sixteen years, and though she didn't have an actual note that said "John sent me," I am sure we were intended to find each other.

*   *   *   *   *

I am not a dog expert of any sort. Every dog I have ever had has been a wonderful mix of various types of dogs, a mutt, as we know them to be. And all of those dogs have been strays, whether we got them from the animal shelter or they simply came to our home and asked to join us. I love strays. I have a habit of attracting them—strays of all sorts, both animal and human. But here I will stick with the canine stray, at least for a while.

I am calling Daisy a border collie, but she is not a purebred by any means. Over the sixteen years she has been with us, she has grown to around thirty pounds. She has a beautiful face and delightful smile. She prances when she walks, and we have always thought she would parade well in a dog show. But we don't know much about dog shows—though Daisy did win Reserve Grand Champion once at the regional fair under our daughter's supervision—and we have never followed through with any of our ideas to start her in agility training.

Daisy definitely has a lot of border collie in her. We aren't sure what other genes may be in there. We do know that she is smart, trainable, loyal, and very connected to us. Those features were what started me thinking about the similarities between Daisy and me.

Over these years Daisy has lived with us, I have been involved in all sorts of self-growth centered on my own codependence. I became aware of some of my issues of overinvolvement with others when my husband stopped drinking and I started attending a twelve-step program for family and friends of alcoholics. Through that program, counseling, reading, and lots of good conversations with "knowing friends," I have been learning a lot about how to find a better balance in my life between focusing on my self and focusing on others.

It was probably that "focusing on others" behavior of Daisy's that first drew my attention to our similarities. It is common for me to be doing something in our house, practically anything, and to look over and see Daisy sitting near me and staring at me. She is watching me ever so carefully, not letting her gaze be diverted by anything. Her big, brown eyes lovingly look at me, and she patiently sits and watches and waits. I do not know what she is waiting for, but my experience with Daisy is that she is waiting for me to notice her, for me to give her my attention, for us to be connected again.

Being such a good codependent my self, I am charmed by her watchful behavior, and I, too, am pleased to once again be connected with my buddy. We are quite a pair.

And that's why I am able to share this book with you—not because I am an expert on dogs or border collies specifically, but because I do know about codependence, and I think both Daisy and I have got it.

M y work on this book has been slow. The idea started in my head over eleven years ago, and then about ten years ago, while on a spring vacation, I wrote out what is now the table of contents for this book. As you can see by reading that table of contents, there are many characteristics that I believe Daisy and I share:

Smart

Devoted

Hardworking

Serving

People Pleasing

Sensitive

Adaptable

Herding

Reactive

Tenacious

Delighted

Big-Hearted

I have gleaned these characteristics through the sixteen years Daisy and I have lived together. Over and over, I am amazed at how often I identify with her behaviors. My daughter has even taken to saying to me at times, "You are such a border collie."

Please know that I speak of these similarities with great endearment. The characteristics that Daisy and I share are often positive qualities that are adaptive for each of us and that bring success and pleasure to our lives. Daisy's herding style is in her breed and is the "work" she does in life, even if I am the main one she herds. Her barking at strangers, even when we reassure her that all is well, is her way of protecting and defending us. Her devotion and watchful eye are welcomed reminders of her loving companionship.

But, as with most things, we can have too much of a good thing.

And so it is true with the characteristics Daisy and I share. And so it is true with the characteristics of codependence. To be loving, kind, thoughtful, giving, involved, helpful, and caring is not bad. In fact, those are valuable features that enrich the world. But we can carry them too far. They can dominate the way we spend our time, the way we run our lives, and the choices we make for ourselves.

Codependence was first identified and named in the field of alcoholism. It was used to describe the partner or the person closest to the alcoholic. This person, the codependent, was seen to respond and to react to the alcoholic in ways that both intentionally and inadvertently contribute to the disease of alcoholism. The codependent was, in fact, a partner to the dependency of the other person on alcohol.

In this early work of identifying and defining codependence, Robin Norwood, in *Women Who Love Too Much*, speaks of the codependent as the co-alcoholic. Norwood explains that the co-alcoholic has developed unhealthy relationship patterns as a result of close involvement with someone with the disease of alcoholism. Those patterns include a need to be needed and persistent efforts to change and/or control others.[2]

And Melody Beattie writes in her landmark book, *Codependent No More*, "A codependent person is one who has let another person's behavior affect him or her, and who is obsessed with controlling that person's behavior."[3]

These were all early, successful attempts to name a psychological condition I would broadly define as having many characteristics that I would precede with the word *over:* overdoing, overgiving, overstating, overresponsible, overcompliant, overcontrolling, overpicky, overloyal. You get the point: Codependent behavior can just be too much. It is over the top. And in this overdone way of life, self is lost.

To this day, codependence remains a loosely defined concept— loosely defined by the standards of the *Diagnostic and Statistical Manual of Mental Disorders* (*DSM-IV*) that we use for diagnostic and treatment purposes in psychology.[4] Codependence is not yet in the *DSM*. Conversations with professionals about this diagnostic situation have revealed that they usually diagnose the individual based on symptoms such as depression and anxiety, which can often be present in the codependent. But no diagnosis yet addresses the intra- and interpersonal dynamics that dominate the codependent's experience.

Thus, we are left to understand it through various definitions well stated by those in recovery as well as by professionals in the fields of mental health and substance abuse.

Just because it is not officially named, though, does not mean we don't know it when we see it. And when we see it, it may look like this . . .

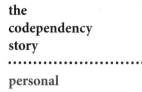
I wasn't born understanding codependency. I didn't even know the word as I entered my professional work as a counselor in 1977. The fields of psychology and substance abuse hardly knew the word, either. What I did know then as I started my career and first marriage was that I had led a fairly successful little life with good grades, a good education, and a good reputation for solid, reliable work. You could count on Nancy. My sorority in college gave me one of the higher awards for leadership, because, I am now sure, I was a steady, reliable, and productive member. Not bad assets.

There were other characteristics about my self as well: I was very much a people pleaser, hated conflict and didn't know how to deal with it, worried about important people leaving me, and was afraid of veering far off the path I thought I was supposed to travel, whether that path was at home or in relationships, school, work, or independent thought.

In 1981 these assorted characteristics only began to start making sense to me as I met the man who was to become my second husband. Independent in thought and action, smart and articulate, this man was truly my "match."

On a subconscious level I had said to my self for several years prior, after my first marriage to my high school sweetheart ended, "You need to meet your match." What I have come to understand about this desire is that I wanted to be with someone who would respectfully press against my will and control and ideas. I could freely, competently, and respectfully press back, and we could learn from each other. This is the sophisticated description that I can offer on paper now and that reflects what I have come to understand as an intuitive desire of mine that I experienced then without my full understanding, a desire greater than anything I could plan or prescribe. But all I knew then was that I wanted to "meet my match."

And "meet my match" I did. Dating an active alcoholic in the early 1980s, the man who was to become my second husband, I fell deeply into my insecure pleasing and worry. But rather than move away from him and all of my uncomfortable feelings, I moved toward them.

My first direct experience with defining codependence occurred around 1986 when this man recommended I buy Robin Norwood's *Women Who Love Too Much: When You Keep Wishing and Hoping He'll Change*. I remember we were shopping in a mall when Monty saw the recently released book on display just outside of a bookstore. Joking, he said, "Maybe you should buy this, Nance." Yes, the origins of my work on codependence came from cooperatively following his indirect advice in order to please him.

An assortment of reactions popped up in me immediately. Remember, I had no self-awareness then about my self and codependence. I thought I was just lovely and charming, but his suggestion set off that worry and insecurity of mine. I thought a couple of things.

First: "How dare he suggest that something is wrong with me! What does he mean by recommending that I buy some type of self-help book?" I felt offended and irritated.

Then I thought, "But I want him to like me, so I'd better show some interest and willingness to consider this book. I'm sure he knows what he is talking about. I don't want to appear stupid or naïve or defensive."

So I did buy the book. I bought a book I knew nothing about in order to please someone else. I bought the book out of my own codependence.

And it has made a world of difference in my life.

As I mentioned previously, the origins of the naming of codependence come from the field of alcoholism. And in the book *Women Who Love Too Much,* Robin Norwood opened my eyes to my self and to the possible relationship between my lostness and the alcoholism in my partner. Perhaps I was the co-alcoholic of which she spoke.

It was all news to me.

We had not yet named alcoholism as an aspect of our relationship, but it is interesting how both my codependence and some meager level of intuition brought me to this new and powerful information, information that helped me to start, but only start, directing the focus to my self.

By 1988 Monty and I were married, had become the parents of Grace, and were a recovering household. I found my way to a twelve-step fellowship by December of that year, still pretty clueless about my part in my relationship problems. I remember going to my first meeting with our three-month-old daughter in my arms, thinking of my self as the wonderfully devoted wife there to help my husband. Charming and gracious, I was there almost in the spirit of attending a social event.

That spirit was short-lived. The relationship difficulties of alcoholism remained, even with the recovery of the alcoholic. In fact, the problems worsened as the absence of alcohol exposed us to raw life.

My twelve-step fellowship does not directly define codependence, but it does offer a place for healing that teaches us to keep the focus on our self and not on others. Codependence deeply wants us to focus on the other person, and this twelve-step prescription is a way of understanding the codependence that brought us into its doors.

I started to pay more attention to my self.

In those early years of recovery I also found Melody Beattie's *Codependent No More,* which has become a classic in its definitions of codependence and treatment ideas. I remember starting to read it in the midst of great tension and discord in our marriage within the first year of recovery. I don't remember what the arguments were about, but I do remember a special day of connecting with *Codependent No More.*

I was scheduled to have our daughter's first studio picture taken. Something went wrong at home. I dressed her up and took her by myself for the photo shoot. She was unhappy with the process, which took too long. Finally, we got a few good pictures and left. I did not want to go home, and since I had put my new book in the car, I headed up to the Blue Ridge Parkway to ride and then read. By the time I got up to the Peaks of Otter, Grace was sound asleep in her car seat. I parked the car in the shade and opened the book. Immediately I found a quotation that suggested that we can only find happiness within our self.

I read on.

Over and over I noticed the mention of control. Robin Norwood advises that we stop managing and controlling others as a part of our recovery.[5] I remember being offended and almost incredulous when I first read this. Me? Controlling? That did not fit my image of my self at all. I thought I was helpful and productive. And then I find that Melody Beattie also says, "We are obsessed with controlling that other person's behavior."[6]

I started to pay attention to my controlling behaviors.

In 1988, as we became parents and as we entered recovery, I also started a job as a counselor in the counseling center of a women's college. Earlier in my counseling career I had already established a specialty in substance abuse, a specialty not based in recovery. How odd to think of my self as specializing in the treatment of substance use when in fact I was living unawares in the middle of alcoholism. From a codependent stance, though, this makes perfect sense in terms of denial, people pleasing, and conflict avoiding on my part, to name a few codependent behaviors.

Nevertheless, substance abuse was one of my specialty areas, and as my recovery progressed, so did my ability to treat it. I became involved in alcohol education for our students, teaching it in classes and in residence hall meetings. As I did so, I learned more about not only the alcoholic, but also the codependent.

The writings of Sharon Wegscheider-Cruse and Janet Woititz have been particularly important to me as I have worked with my self and others. I use their material so often and richly that I have come to think of what they produced as classics in our fields. Among her accomplishments, Sharon Wegscheider-Cruse outlined the roles performed in addicted families: Dependent, Enabler, Hero, Scapegoat, Lost Child, and Mascot.[7] How interesting it was to me to understand my behaviors in terms of these roles. I learned not only the characteristics of the roles, but also that our rigid attachment to the roles we take on is as much of the problem for our self as anything. I found that I am basically a hero with mascot features. Being a hero has its advantages: we perform pretty well in life; people can depend on us; we are reliable and productive. But to be stuck in this role with constant high expectations and heavy demands for my self is a rough way to live in the long run. It is exhausting and never-ending, frustrating for me at times, and it can be too much for others.

I started paying attention to my hero way of life.

Among her accomplishments, Janet Woititz gave an excellent look at the characteristics of adult children of alcoholics in *Adult Children of Alcoholics*.[8] I found this book as I was developing my self as well as programs for the college students with whom I was working. Though I was not raised in an alcoholic home, I was struck by the similarities between adult children of alcoholics and those of us who have developed codependent characteristics as a result of other childhood experiences. In a later, expanded version of this book, Woititz herself comments on this applicability of her material to the full range of family dysfunction, including anyone who grew up with addiction in any form.

So what was I finding true for me? Well, let's put it this way: I have at least eight of the thirteen characteristics Woititz describes. My characteristics include judging my self without mercy, difficulty having fun, taking my self very seriously, difficulty with intimate relationships, constantly seeking approval and affirmation, being super-responsible, and being extremely loyal. I am pleased to say that I have succeeded at moderating all of these characteristics and their effects on my life, but suffice it to say, when I found this information in the late 1980s I was amazed at this view of my self and new way to understand me.

I started paying attention to my serious, overdone self.

In this same time period of the late 1980s and early 1990s I came upon another useful clinical document about codependence. Timmen Cermak's book *Diagnosing and Treating Co-Dependence* presents the characteristics of codependence in the form used by the *DSM-IV*. Cermak also presents the diagnostic criteria for his proposed "Co-Dependent Personality Disorder."[9] This work is theoretical and built from clinical and anecdotal information as opposed to research; however, I found it to be an interesting early attempt to say that these codependent behaviors can really be a problem for people and need to receive professional consideration and help.

Cermak's criteria for the "Co-Dependent Personality Disorder" include

- self-esteem dependent on the ability to control others;
- needs of others consistently placed ahead of one's own needs;
- anxiety and boundary distortions around getting close to and separating from others; and
- unclear boundaries between self and others.

Cermak acknowledges that many people have some of these characteristics, and that these characteristics become a diagnosable problem only when they are extreme enough to interfere with their functioning in work and/or relationships. That is where the differences start showing up between simply doing good, being kind, and offering help and doing damage to self and others.

I started paying attention to ways my helping was hurting my self and others.

In the spring of 1990 I wrote my own paper, "Diagnosing Codependence." I was a graduate student taking classes to complete my license as a professional counselor. The class was a seminar in psychopathology. I continued to be interested in the topic of codependence, and used this class assignment as an opportunity to write some of my compiled ideas.

Like Cermak, I was interested in working with the professional format of the *DSM-IV*. I organized my criteria for the proposed "Codependent Personality Disorder" under the umbrella of other-centeredness. "The essential feature of this disorder is a pervasive pattern of other-centeredness . . . . The person may sacrifice his or her own needs for those of others, think obsessively about and try unreasonably to control the behavior of others, and allow his or her identity and self-esteem to be governed by the opinions and feelings of others." [10]

Other-centeredness: I was learning this in my twelve-step program. I was learning this through readings. I was learning this by working with others. I was learning this by observing my self.

I kept paying attention to my other-centeredness.

In 1993, recognizing my continuing need to add to my recovery program, I attended a workshop with Toby Rice Drews as the presenter. I did not know her previous work but was drawn directly to her session based on her recently released book *Getting Them Sober, Volume 4: Separations and Healings.* [11] At that time I continued to feel lost in my primary relationships. I could feel anywhere from guilty to depressed, and often acted in obsessive ways, seeking affection, reassurance, and validation—most of which I did not find through my seeking. Sometimes I was a functioning mess. It is powerful for me to read my journals from that time and hear my stuck and lost self. Recovery is an amazing process.

My participation in Toby's workshop not only taught me much, but it also opened the door to look at my pain, my history, my behaviors, my choices. My progress was slow and painful and not even clearly visible then.

One of the many themes of my work was my learning to see the reality of things, especially in my marriage. In the language of recovery, this is called breaking through denial. I was able to see the reality of my language and behaviors and my husband's language and behaviors. I learned that illusions are a big part of what keeps us stuck, and what a big hole that was for me.

I started paying attention to my illusions.

Through this work and my twelve-step involvement I started to put some other pieces of recovery in place for my self as well. Detaching and setting healthy boundaries emerged as concrete areas of personal work, along with facing illusions. My awareness of these specific areas of work developed in the following way:

Sometime in 1994 I was finishing an appointment with a client in my private practice. We were standing inside my office with the door closed, saying good-bye, when the client asked a most profound question. She said, "I understand what you mean about getting emotional distance from my husband, but how do you do that?"

It is common in therapy for the more powerful, deep material to come to the surface late in a session. Consciously or unconsciously, this is what can happen. Yet for a therapist to be effective, it is important to maintain healthy boundaries, including those of time, which means to stop on time regardless of the content unless it involves life-threatening information. I knew this, but at the same time I was struck by her question.

Pushing the edges of our time boundaries, I continued the session a bit longer. I did not invite her to sit down, but I grabbed a piece of paper, sat on the edge of my desk chair, and jotted down six to eight ideas that immediately came to my mind on how to create some emotional distance. The ideas came quickly and easily. They were close to my work and my heart. I copied the list and gave her the original to study for homework.

As the same clinical day went on, I was amazed at how many times that list of ideas about creating emotional distance was applicable. A woman dealing with a demanding mother-in-law, a woman unsure about her relationship with her boss, a man left by his girlfriend all could use this information, and I copied the same list for them.

At this time I was also working with college students, and I quickly started to see how handy this list of ideas was in helping students deal with emerging independence, family-of-origin dysfunction, and significant relationships—any clinical issue that involved development and assertion of self.

The list became longer as we all worked with this material together. The list became long enough that I could divide it into sections. I identified four areas of work:

- Facing Illusions
- Detaching
- Setting Healthy Boundaries
- Developing Spirituality

The word *disentangle* emerged for this work, and this now-three-page, four-section handout was entitled "Ideas on How to Disentangle." We started holding "Disentangle" groups. The only requirement for membership was a relationship entanglement, past or present. Adult children of alcoholics, people loving too much, codependents, people afraid of abandonment, people pleasers, and conflict avoiders all came together to work on the core issues of self.

I was paying more and more attention to my need for self-development.

By 1996 I realized that I could write a book from all of this "Disentangle" work. In fact, I realized that the book was already written; I just needed to put it on paper. Not only did I have the handout as my book outline, but I also had many hours of active conversations with people, individually and in groups, that clarified and expanded the information. So over the course of several years I wrote *Disentangle: When You've Lost Your Self in Someone Else.*[12]

The book has continued to be a very active project for me. Not only has it given me the opportunity to do many workshops, meet wonderful people, and travel to new places, it has also provided me with the continuing opportunity for my own growth and recovery. How can I teach something that I do not know from the inside out? Recently I was writing an advertisement for a codependence camp for counselors, and I thought to write as the lead-in line:

The more I know about my self, the more I can help others.

Now, that statement can sound codependent if I am not careful. I am not doing this personal work so that I can help others. I am doing this personal work so I can have peace, serenity, and better relationships with my self and with others. If and when I am able to gain these things for my self, then my being able to share and help others with these issues will be a spiritual bonus.

Yes, it will be a spiritual bonus.

This leads me to say a bit more about my story of codependency and spirituality.

As I was writing about the evolution of the four sections of *Disentangle*, I realized I had mentioned illusions, detaching, and boundaries previously, but added spirituality as the fourth section without any explanation. This realization prompted me to look more carefully at that part of my story.

The development of my spirituality has been sweet and soothing. I credit my involvement with the twelve-step programs as the foundational source of my evolving spirituality. Through the programs I learned to sort what I can and cannot control, and I made a decision to believe in a power greater than my self to which I let go of those things I cannot control. So much of codependence is about trying to control what we have no control over, usually other people, places, and things. For me, developing this belief in a power/force/flow greater than me allows me to create a safety net for my self as I do this challenging work of letting go of what I can't control or change.

Not only do I choose to believe in this safety net, but also I choose to trust it. I have learned to trust it in this way: Once I have let go, what happens may or may not be what I thought was best or what I wanted. I trust that what happens is what is supposed to happen. I have even gotten to the point where I can be excited to see what does or does not happen after I have removed my false grasp on a person or situation. I call this living in the flow—doing my part as fully and honestly as possible and then letting go to the bigger, broader aspects of life. Moment by moment, I repeat this process over the course of a day.

Do my part and let go. Do my part and let go.

I notice my natural use of the phrase *moment by moment.* Being in the moment has become an important part of my spirituality. Living in the present and coming back to the present are things I have learned through my story as well, and I credit my study and practice of mindfulness for this.

In 1996, I took a series of mindfulness-based stress-reduction and relaxation classes at the University of Virginia Medical School. These classes were modeled after the original program of the same name created and run by Jon Kabat-Zinn at the University of Massachusetts and fully presented in *Full Catastrophe Living.*[13] I had learned about Kabat-Zinn's work with mindfulness and had been interested in studying with him when I found out about this offer that was more convenient for me.

The series of eight classes taught the use of the deep breath, gentle *hatha* yoga, and the body scan as formal ways to learn to attend to the present moment. The classes also directed us toward ways to informally practice these skills of coming back to the present moment over and over through the course of our days.

Since taking that series of classes, I have been offering similar classes through my private practice. I call my classes "Mindful Living."

I am often working on mindfully living. To me this means quieting my thoughts and noticing the sounds and sensations of what I am experiencing at that moment. To me it means noticing when I am judging something or someone and being able to stop that and just allow what is. To me it means noticing my breath and following it and settling into it as my internal thermostat is then naturally calmed and quieted. To me it means opening my self to what I am defending against, and to that end it opens me to so much more, including my spirituality.

As I quiet and open, I can let go of what I think has to happen, of what I think is the best solution, of what I want to be true. In this opening, I also open to a power greater than my self, and I relax as I lighten my unnecessarily heavy load and let the flow of life proceed without my trying to dam it up.

I am learning that mindfulness brings me back to my true self, and my true self is, among many things, spiritual.

Since 2000 I have been trying to further understand and apply all of these wonderful lessons from the previous twelve years. Life has been both hard and good. I have had daily opportunities to be either in the solution or in the problem, as the twelve-step programs say. I spend time in both. I hope I am spending less time in the problem, and I believe I am based on increased serenity, a greatly enhanced ability to listen to my self, and improved skills in self-expression and assertion.

My individual work through meetings, conversations with others on this path, readings, workshops, retreats, and writings has helped me to continue to work on me.

Opportunities to present the material I offer in *Disentangle* have also helped me to grow and to help others in their growth. For this I am very grateful.

In the preparation of these presentations, I decided to revisit what the professionals have been researching and writing about codependence in recent years. Yes, I know my story and its sources, as I have just told it to you. I felt like it also was important to know and share the most current research data available as I have gone out into the world with my work.

In many ways codependence has come up through the ranks of self-help, which has taught us much about what codependency is and how to recover from it. For this I am also grateful. Codependence is a very real style of being and of interacting and merits the serious attention of both laypeople and professionals. The more the treatment providers and academic researchers can come together with definition and clarity on this topic, the better we all will be, and I do mean all of us.

So off to a university library I went, and here is what I found.

A s of 2012, we still have not made significant progress in studying, defining, and formalizing codependence in our professional world. Individual studies certainly are being done, and efforts to develop an assessment tool that is reliable and valid for codependence are being made. But no great conclusions have been drawn that help us all to agree on a definition of and treatment strategies for codependence. The writers and researchers I read have frequently commented on this observation as well.

In a chapter entitled "Treating the Partners of Substance Abusers," Elizabeth Zelvin states, "The spouses and partners of alcohol and drug abusers constitute an almost forgotten population in the treatment of alcohol and other drug (AOD) dependence . . . . A recent literature search yielded only a handful of new articles in 2002 and 2003 on spouses or partners of people with alcoholic or other kinds of substance problems in the United States."[14]

Zelvin continues, "The partner of the AOD-dependent individual must be treated as a primary client who needs and deserves help for his or her own sake."[15]

Related to this lack of research are controversial issues with the use of the word *codependent* and ways codependency should be approached and treated. Researchers on this topic acknowledge that the word *codependent* is both popular and overused, that the term does not reflect the use of careful scientific methods to define and apply, and that more assessment and evaluation are needed to effectively identify, diagnose, and treat these individuals.

Looking at codependence from a gender perspective, writers describe ways in which the concept of codependence has not been viewed as an effect of living in a patriarchal society, an effect especially seen in women. Janice Haaken offers that the oppression of women has significantly contributed to the caregiving role taken on by women, and rather than see the tendency to become very involved with the needs of others as a sickness, it is important to see those behaviors within the context of the social worlds within which the individual has grown and lived.[16] Elizabeth Zelvin adds support to this observation, stating that society, too, must be considered as a force creating and maintaining what we are calling codependence.[17]

From this gender perspective we see that in a male-dominated society, women have learned to be the caregivers and people pleasers, the compliant and submissive ones, the ones without a voice and even, perhaps, without a known self.

Considering these literature findings and important controversies, the following is how I choose, at this time, to understand and treat what we call codependence.

*   *   *   *   *

My literature review yielded a continuing variety of ways to define codependency and to explain its origins. My interpretation of this material has involved integrating the ideas rather than declaring one right/one wrong or one possible/one not. Zelvin, too, states, "Codependent pathology is independent of any single relationship. It may come from a dysfunctional family of origin, the chemically dependent relationship, existing social norms, or from all of these. In women especially, it may represent a distortion of the healthy need to connect."[18]

In working to integrate our various understandings of codependence, I found that the given definitions could be categorized as having an individual emphasis, a family systems emphasis, and a social/cultural/political emphasis. To illustrate the interrelationship of these definitions, I developed this diagram:

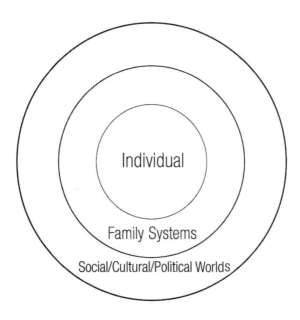

In the center of the diagram is the individual person. That is you or me. We live within a family system, whatever form that may take, and we come from a family-of-origin system, again whatever form that may have taken. Our family systems live within social/cultural/political worlds. Each of these outer layers has profound effects on the individual it surrounds. To understand codependence in the individual without seeing these layers of influence on them is incomplete.

Let's look at definitions that focus on the **Individual** first.

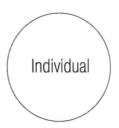

I have already presented both Robin Norwood's and Melody Beattie's early definitions of codependence that present the codependent as a person strongly affected by someone else's behavior and wanting to control that other person.

Codependents Anonymous (CoDA) was established in 1986. Adapting the Twelve Steps and Twelve Traditions from Alcoholics Anonymous (AA), this organization describes codependence in terms of patterns and characteristics rather than a formal definition or list of criteria to be met. The patterns and characteristics include denial, low self-esteem, compliance, control, and avoidance. CoDA provides an excellent list of behaviors under each of these characteristics for self-evaluation (http://www.coda.org).

In recent years, Greg Dear, Clare Roberts, and Lois Lange have been working to develop a professional assessment tool for codependence: the Holyoake Codependency Index. As an essential part of this work, they analyzed eleven of the most widely cited published definitions of codependency and identified four core defining features of codependency, which they presented in their article "Defining

Codependency: A Thematic Analysis of Published Definitions":[19]

- **External focusing**
- **Self-sacrificing**
- **Interpersonal control**
- **Emotional suppression**

Here are the ways Dear and Roberts define each of these elements*:[20]

- **External focusing** refers to focusing one's attention on the behaviors, opinions, and expectations of other people and then fitting one's own behavior to those expectations or opinions to obtain approval and esteem.
- **Self-sacrificing** refers to neglecting one's own needs to focus on meeting the needs of other people.
- **Interpersonal control** reflects an entrenched belief in one's capacity to fix other people's problems and control their behavior.
- **Emotional suppression** refers to the deliberate suppression, or limited conscious awareness, of one's emotions until they become overwhelming.

It is interesting to see how this scientifically derived list of behaviors associated with codependence matches the list generated and used by CoDA and others. As we study these various ways codependence is defined in the individual, we start to see the individual as focused on other(s), strongly affected by other(s), and not sure how to and/or unable to act on his or her own behalf. These are broad, general themes, but nevertheless they create an important picture of the individual for whom codependence is a problem. The individual is externally oriented, looking outside of his or her self for ideas, fulfillment, and validation. The individual's sense of self is dependent on these external people, places, and things. Several researchers highlight this dynamic as well.

Barbara Yoder describes co-alcoholics and those who live with other forms of addiction and/or dysfunction as giving up on their own lives, as living their lives through someone else in order to please others or escape the pain of their difficult family situations. In so doing, these individuals are obscuring their own identity.[21]

Teri Loughead also looks at this sense of self in her study of codependence. She theorizes that codependence is an underlying dynamic of addiction. She describes addiction, in whatever form, as an attempt to establish a desired feeling state. The individual's feeling state, she maintains, is affected by his or her sense of self. When our sense of self feels weak, threatened, inadequate, depressed, or anxious, then addictive behaviors may be used to help us feel more whole and less disturbed.[22]

In terms of codependence specifically, this is addressing, again, the pattern of being dependent on things outside of our self, especially on others, to change and improve our feeling state and our ability to function, rather than helping our self from within. So when things coming at us aren't so good, we may feel fragmented and lost. Our ability to function then declines, and psychological symptoms of depression and anxiety may emerge.

What we want to do is to cultivate that center circle, that circle I have labeled "Individual." We will talk more about this cultivation throughout this book, but for now I want to emphasize that I see the treatment of codependence as self-development. This brief review of some of the literature on codependence is repeatedly describing this loss of self, this abdication of self to others, this dependence on things outside of our self for our well-being. Our recovery involves turning this around and bringing our focus to our self and then helping that self to become well and strong. And you can do that.

Referring back to my diagram explaining definitions and sources of codependence, let's look at the **Family Systems** layer surrounding the Individual.

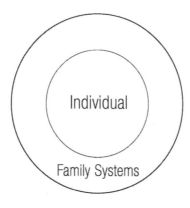

Even in the previous definitions, we have already seen references to the family system of the individual with codependent behaviors. Certainly individuals may have within themselves tendencies toward codependence that stem from their mood and/or personality features, but it is hard to separate those personal sources from the past and present influences of the individuals' family systems.

Layne Prest and Howard Protinsky propose that we not look at codependence as a reaction in an individual to another individual, but rather see that family members are responding to the dysfunctional system in which they live. Further, they maintain that rather than develop a list of characteristics of the codependent, we should study the characteristics of the codependent's family system. They are interested in both the family of origin of the individuals and their current family systems.[23]

What do we mean by "family system"?

Well, simply put, each of us is a member of a family. Our

first family is the family with which we grew up. We call that our family of origin. Then, as we become adults, most of us develop yet another family, which we can call our current family. This may include a significant other as well as our children. It may also still include members of our family of origin.

We use the word *system* here because of the interrelationship between each of the members in a family. How one person in the family acts, feels, and thinks affects how other family members act, feel, and think.

Some researchers and therapists have studied family systems extensively. Here are several ways we can look at the meaning of codependence from a family perspective.

In early work in this field of codependence, Robert Subby and John Friel wrote about the characteristics of codependents' families. They spoke of this interrelationship between family members in terms of rules we learned as we grew up. They maintain that the way we operate as adults is affected by the rules we learned from our family of origin. Some of the family rules that contribute to codependence include not talking about feelings or problems, indirect communication among family members, and messages to be strong, good, perfect, and not selfish. Additionally important rules involve making the family proud and not causing problems.[24]

As Loughead examined these rules further, she commented on the consequences to the individual of such rules: an inaccurate perception of reality; problems with trust, relating to others, and handling emotions; and a damaged image of self.[25]

In other words, as we look back at the characteristics of the codependent individual presented earlier, we see how these dynamics in the family system cause the person to have no sense of self or an inaccurate sense of self as a result of looking outside of his or her self for how to be, trying to please, and not speaking honestly. This descriptive list echoes some of the defining features of codependence named by Dear and Roberts: external focusing, self-sacrificing, and emotional suppression.

In addition to family rules, family roles are important in understanding an individual's style of relating and coping in the world. In 1989, Sharon Wegscheider-Cruse carried this work on the relationship of the family to the individual further by describing frequently defined roles taken on by members of a family system in which the above rules were likely active: Dependent, Enabler, Hero, Scapegoat, Lost Child, and Mascot.[26]

These roles were defined with the alcoholic system in mind and in experience. We have learned, however, that these roles can be taken on in any family system in which the functioning of the family is limited by the rules described by Subby and Friel and/or a family system in which other forms of addiction, compulsions, illnesses, or extreme behaviors are present.

Looking at these roles from the family systems perspective, what happens is that the needs and behaviors of one person throw off the balance of the family system, and, whether they realize it or not, each person takes on a role to restore that illusory balance. And most of the time they do not realize they have taken on their roles.

In the classical use of these roles, the Dependent is the person who has the obvious addiction/compulsion/extreme behavior, and this is usually one of the parents.

The partner of that Dependent often takes on the role of Enabler, feeling powerless over the Dependent and reacting by taking on too much responsibility for practically everything. This overresponsibility is an effort to hold things together and to control what he or she cannot control.

And then there are the roles taken on by the children in this out-of-balance family system.

The Hero is often the firstborn child. Heroes are high-achieving individuals. They are the ones who usually do things right. They work hard. They accomplish much. They make the family proud of them. They can be counted on. They gather positive attention that helps to increase the feelings of self-worth for their suffering family systems.

The Scapegoat is often the second-born child. Scapegoats present as troubled in some way. Perhaps they have problems with the law, with substances, with school. They are the ones the family looks to and says, "Everything would be just fine if [this child] would just act right." They are acting out their hurt. Their self-destructive ways draw negative attention and may help to move the negative focus away from the Dependent.

The Lost Child may be the third child. Lost children like to spend time alone. They may be found in their room or some quiet, private place escaping from the out-of-balance dynamics of their family. They enjoy solitary activities such as reading or creating imaginary play. Their social isolation provides relief for the family, but interpersonal deficits for the child.

The Mascot is frequently the last child. Mascots try to restore balance to the family system through humor and entertainment. They may make people laugh and have a bit of fun. They may clown, tell amusing stories, or simply divert conflict into lively and lighter antics and conversations.

There are several things I want to say about these roles.

First, these roles are well described and often extremely accurate. When I am getting to know a client, it is not uncommon for me to guess his or her birth order simply based on the characteristics he or she is telling me about his or her self.

Second, though these roles are presented in this order and frequently do fall in this birth order in a family system, they do not have to be taken on in this given birth order. A second-born may be the Hero. The first child may be the Lost Child. But when these exceptions are present, there is usually an understandable family-dynamics reason for the variation.

Third, a family system does not have to have four children to assume all of these roles. All four roles will be assumed by however many children there are in a family system. So if there are two children, they will each take on roles until all of the roles are played out. You see, the family needs all of these roles to be in action in order to try to keep the precarious and false balance of the disturbed family system.

The problem for us as individuals is not these roles themselves. Each serves a purpose and has a functional range. The problem comes when we become locked in a role. We believe we always have to be the responsible one. We know we are the "black sheep." We believe we just need to once again retreat and be alone. Not only do we believe that we must maintain our role, but other members of our family system do not know us in any way other than the role we have assumed and played out so well, and they expect us to continue as we always have.

As Wegscheider-Cruse points out, there are consequences to the extreme behaviors of each role. The Hero can become compulsively driven. The Scapegoat can become self-destructive. The Lost Child can develop social isolation. The Mascot can remain immature and may have emotional illness.

What we want for our healthy self-development is to recognize the role(s) we have taken on in our family system, notice them in our daily life, and become flexible about whether we want to play that role here and now or not. We do not want to have our role(s) be the only way we operate and the only way people know and respond to us.

While all this information about family systems so far has been at our family of origin, what we know is that if we are not aware of our original family's rules and roles, we will self-select those same or similar rules and roles in the family systems we create for our self as adults. Why? Because that is what we know and what we do and how we handle our self. That is the self we know, whether we realize it or not.

Yes, there are individuals who grow up in more balanced homes and who do not identify with either the rules or the roles presented here. But you are reading this book because something is out of balance for you. I offer a couple of thoughts here about how your family system may be affecting you.

First, I have found through my clinical and personal work that we often have not been aware of how our family operated and what our reactions were to that system. We knew, for example, that someone drank too much or someone wasn't home much, but we came to see that as just the way it was. Some people even came to see it as normal, as they had no other frame of reference with which to compare their family with others. We have no awareness of the imbalance that may be present. It isn't until we start trying to understand our self that we look in more detail and with more information at our family of origin. Then these roles and relationships begin to make more sense.

I have also found instances where these roles and rules were not in a person's immediate family of origin. Perhaps there was no one with overt problems or extreme behaviors that threw off the family system balance. In such cases what I find sometimes is that an individual's current behavior (e.g., codependent behavior style) was modeled for him or her by a parent. It is likely that that parent grew up in an out-of-balance family system and thus took on the role of helping, pleasing, and being overresponsible. In the parent's adult life, he or she has maintained that role and the child/children have learned it from him or her.

For example, someone I know grew up with a father who was a minister. When I first met this person, he described his father as someone he idolized, selfless and always giving to others. Not only did he have his church responsibilities, but he volunteered for many community activities and was almost always gone from home. He presented this not only as admirable, but as desirable for him as well. He stated that he makes decisions that he believes his father, too, would have made about how to treat people and about being generous and helpful.

This same individual, however, has been unhappily married for twenty years to an active alcoholic. Unable to leave his spouse or set healthy boundaries with her, he struggles with wanting to leave her and wanting to take good care of her. Poor boundaries and excessive caretaking of others modeled by his father have taken strong root in him. And though his father's behaviors are of merit to a degree, clearly they can go too far and be taught to others in unintended and unhelpful ways.

So whatever our family history may have been, I find it useful to look at our self in that context—to see rules, roles, and relationships, and to see how we were treated and how what we learned then affects us now.

There are many other important writings on the ways our family system affects us. Family system theorists and practitioners have created clear and useful ways to understand and treat these out-of-balance family dynamics. Over the past thirty years, a great deal of psychological research and writing has been done on childhood development, looking at issues of health as well as the effects of abuse and trauma. Additional family system readings may be useful to you as you work to understand who you are and how you want to be.

To complete this picture of codependence, let's once again look at my diagram illustrating sources of codependence and study the third layer surrounding the Individual and Family layers: **Social/Cultural/Political Worlds.**

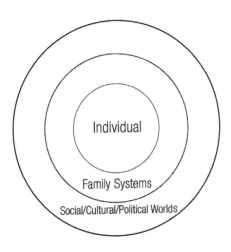

This layer is broad and incorporates many more external aspects of an individual's life that affect who he or she is. This is true for all of us. We have each been influenced by the values and beliefs of our cultures, our churches, our schools, our governments. Family roles can be defined by culture. The way we treat each other can be learned through our religions. Our experiences in school can have a significant impact on our sense of self. The way we are responded to by our governments can affect our sense of autonomy and empowerment.

Codependent behaviors can certainly have roots in these social/cultural/political influences.

Several writers have helped me to see the importance of understanding this third layer's effect on each individual.

Haaken makes some clear and strong points about the influences of societal processes on what we call codependence. She explains that though the women's movement initiated in the late 1960s helped women to have new and expanded opportunities in the workforce, it did not liberate them from the traditional roles of caregiving. She states that seeing codependence as something that is wrong with the woman is moving backward from the progress of the women's movement. Being a caregiving woman is woven into our social and cultural ways and is not to be viewed as a sickness of the individual.

Haaken further argues against seeing codependence simply as the result of rules in a dysfunctional family, and she suggests that we are overusing the disease model in working with family dysfunction. Haaken is concerned that we are pathologizing the individual and his or her family system without looking beyond them to this third layer I am describing. She believes that it is important for us to see those family rules and the dynamics within a family that we call dysfunctional as extensions of historical and societal processes that involve traditional roles, expectations, and power inequalities.[27]

In other words, in order to have a more complete picture of the meaning and sources of codependence, we need to look beyond the individual and his or her family system. The individual and his or her family have been profoundly affected by the social world in which they live, and to not acknowledge this and to not study this is to not offer the individual all the pieces he or she needs in order to create effective changes for his or her growth.

In her chapter on "Treating the Partners of Substance Abusers," Zelvin credits Anne Wilson Schaef for helping to highlight the role of society in creating and perpetuating addiction and codependency. Schaef brings the disease concept back into play but explains that codependence is a product of a disease process that involves our social systems, which she calls the addictive process.[28]

In describing this disease process, Shaef offers characteristics that she believes can be found in our social institutions, including schools, churches, and government. Some of those characteristics include dishonesty, control, perfectionism, self-centeredness, not dealing with feelings honestly, and looking outside self for validation.[29]

This list, which has many similarities to the lists of codependent behaviors, suggests that what we are studying as codependence is, in fact, prevalent in the very fabric of our daily lives through the social institutions in which we live and participate.

So how do I propose we use this third layer of influences in understanding an individual's codependence? Just as we did with the second layer that examines the family influences—we invite the individual to look at the social, gender, cultural, ethnic, and religious factors that he or she has been taught directly or by example. We look at how those factors have contributed to his or her loss of self. And then, we sort what the individual can and does want to change within this context of his or her family and social worlds.

If the individual wants to learn to think more independently, we work on that.

If the individual wants to speak his or her thoughts and feelings directly, we work on that.

If the individual is doing things not true for him or her, we work on that.

If the individual is tired of trying to please others, we work on that.

If the individual is trying to control what he or she can't, we work on that.

As we do this work, we are bumping into family and social structures that can be anywhere from disapproving to controlling. But we are doing so with more awareness of the total self. And on we go, as best we can, always working toward a healthy connection with self and then gaining a strengthened self that can relate to these family and social worlds in ways that work better, at least for the individual seeking self-change.

In our so doing, perhaps the world will be changed, too—systems being what they are, with one change affecting the entire system.

In the spirit of this book and my work, I will return our focus to our work on our self. Let's get out of the library and go to the workshop classroom.

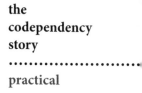

the codependency story

···························

practical

S hortly after I finished writing my first book, *Disentangle: When You've Lost Your Self in Someone Else,* I realized that I could easily offer workshops on its material. That material, in fact, had been largely developed in group counseling settings from the beginning. So I was used to presenting, discussing, dissecting, and explaining many of its concepts with other interested people.

I started offering workshops through my private practice. This work then expanded to offering workshops at conferences and to creating and running what my colleague and I call "Codependence Camp" twice a year. In all of these settings I have been developing ways to help people understand codependent behaviors. I am always interested in trying to study and explain codependence from something other than just a list of behaviors. I am a visual learner, and to that end I have naturally created some diagrams and visual tools to help explain codependent dynamics.

I use the word *dynamics* here, as I write about ways to understand codependence, because I see codependence not only as an attribute—e.g., people pleaser, conflict avoider—but also as an action, as a behavior in time and space. The more we can become aware of our behaviors that entangle us and others, the more we can make active choices about how far to go with those behaviors or whether to continue them at all.

Here is a list of some of these dynamics. In some ways they are similar to the definitions of codependence I have been presenting in this book; however, here I invite you to see these descriptions as **active behaviors** that we can bring into our awareness so as to change as needed and as desired:

- Looking outside of self
- Focusing on the other person
- Doing for others what they could do for themselves
- Doing many things that involve the word *over* as the prefix:
- Overcommitting
- Overextending
- Overfunctioning
- Reacting
- Disconnecting from true feelings
- Disregarding others' boundaries
- Disregarding your own boundaries
- Trying to control things you cannot control
- Forgetting spirituality

With these dynamics in mind, I offer three conceptual tools in diagram form to help us understand codependent behaviors. Each of these conceptual tools—**a balance scale, circles, and a continuum**—offers a mental picture we can use to help us gauge the extent of our loss of self in someone else. These diagrams have all emerged from my presentations and have proven to be useful ways to think about this process of developing a healthy balance between self and others.

With that said, the first practical picture is one of a **balance scale:**

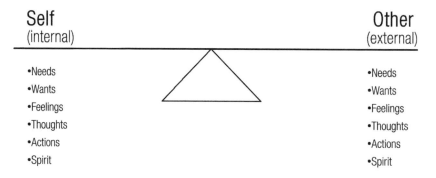

Self (internal)	Other (external)
•Needs	•Needs
•Wants	•Wants
•Feelings	•Feelings
•Thoughts	•Thoughts
•Actions	•Actions
•Spirit	•Spirit

In some ways the lesson of this balance scale is straightforward: we should make sure to keep a healthy balance between our focus on our self and our focus on other(s). Let's look at this in a bit more detail.

You will notice that the ends of the scale are marked not only with "Self" and "Other," but also with "internal" under "Self" and "external" under "Other." As we have already established through definitions, codependent behaviors involve much focusing outside of our self (external): attending to the needs and feelings of others, trying to guess the thoughts and feelings of others, planning for them, doing for them, accommodating them, perhaps to the extent of abandoning our self.

We may not even be aware of the extent to which we have loaded the balance scale, or seesaw, so that the "Other" end is way down while our end of "Self" is flying high. We have not considered our own needs, feelings, thoughts, hopes, and dreams (internal). As someone said so well in a twelve-step meeting after describing a vacation decision, "Where was *I* in the formula?" She was remarking about how everyone else had expressed their feelings and wants about a situation, but she had failed to do so for her self.

As we are looking outside of our self to read and respond and react to the other person, we want to notice if we are also listening to our self. It is so easy to let the balance be off in favor of the other person if we are not attentive to our self as well.

This self-attending can be difficult. Even after we have tuned in to our self, we sometimes don't know what we hear and need. Even once we are able to know more about what we might need and want, we are sorely challenged to know how to express it and take action on it.

Fear not. The Tales and Lessons that follow are written to help you with all of these self-attending tasks. For the present, I am inviting you to see this focusing on self and on others as an active balancing act that requires awareness, a commitment to self, and behavioral changes—all of which keep us from leaving our self up in the air.

The second conceptual diagram uses **circles.** The pictures below help us understand unhealthy and healthy relationships:

Relationships

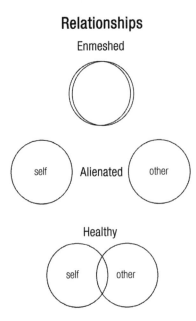

Enmeshed

self Alienated other

Healthy

self other

Consider each circle to be a person. For the sake of this introductory description, the circles are the same size and have the same type of line defining them. In more individualized work, the individual's circles may be smaller or larger in size, depending on his or her sense of self and boundaries, or the line defining the circle may be broken or bold, again depending on the individual's sense of self.

In the first picture, the circles are overlapping to the extent that there is little to no part of each circle that stands alone. The two circles, or people, are eclipsing each other. When these two circles are locked into this formation, we call this *enmeshment*. Neither person has a healthy, separate sense of self, and when either person makes an effort to separate, the other person reacts in a way to restore this level of enmeshment.

Enmeshment can present in various ways. Examples include a relationship in which neither is able to go anywhere without the other person; one person is not free to dress, think, or participate in his or her own activities without the permission of the other; or love and acceptance are conditional on acting or being a specific way. Individual freedom is sacrificed for maintenance of the relationship, sometimes at almost any cost.

The second picture shows the two circles or people completely separate, with no shared selves. As was true in the first picture, these circles remain static. They do not change their basic relationship, which is to never come together in meaningful ways. We call this an *alienated relationship*.

An alienated relationship can present in various ways. Examples include a relationship in which the two individuals are unable and/or unwilling to safely share who they are and what they think, feel, and want. They may share living spaces and a family, and yet still operate in a guarded way so that their self is protected. There may be numerous reasons for this self-protection, including real danger or fear of enmeshment. The costs of this alienation include loneliness and lack of self-growth.

The third picture shows the circles or people overlapping some, yet not completely. In this case, the individuals are able to both share themselves and keep a separate sense of self. We call this a *healthy relationship.*

This diagram of a healthy relationship does not remain static. Rather, it is dynamic, as the individuals are able to move toward or away from each other as needed and desired. Remember, each circle or person has its own boundaries. These two circles can intersect and cross each other as much as is *mutually* agreed upon. So the circles can range from nearly completely overlapped to completely separate depending on the expressed needs of each person and mutual respect between them.

This healthy relationship is dynamic. It allows for change and flow. It is dependent on having two individuals aware of their separateness and togetherness and wanting to foster their self *and* their relationship in this way.

A healthy relationship can present in various ways. Examples include a relationship in which the individuals come together, express their separate thoughts, feelings, and needs, and then respond to each other in the most mutually beneficial way. Obviously this does not mean that either gets his or her way all of the time. Compromise and letting go become an active part of this picture, with not an abdication of self in the process, but a strengthening gained from feeling heard and understood by both our self and the other person.

As you study these circles, perhaps you are already identifying with some aspects of either the circles themselves or the nature of the relationship between the circles: *enmeshed, alienated, healthy.* Maybe your circle is big or small. Maybe its borders are smooth or more like dotted lines. Maybe you are the one who fosters enmeshment, who crosses the other person's boundaries and holds on for dear life. Or maybe the boundaries of your circle are repeatedly battered and invaded, and your very self is challenged and diminished. All of these observations are important foundations for your healthy self-development.

Remember, you are establishing groundwork here by studying these three conceptual tools. And so, as you bring your self to interactions with others, you may want to bring these circles to mind.

Giving/Fixing/Caretaking

OK	Going Too Far
•Make offers <u>within your resources</u> ($, time, energy)	•Make offers <u>outside</u> of your resources and carry them out (causing debt, exhaustion, losses)
•Make offer/<u>accept</u> the other person's acceptance or rejection of your offer	•<u>Force</u> your offer on the other person, insist
•Make suggestion(s) and <u>leave them alone</u>	•<u>Insist</u> upon your suggestions and/or actually carry them out for the other person

The title of the diagram speaks for itself: the continuum is offered to help determine where one is on this line of behaviors related to giving and fixing and caretaking. Of course, in looking at definitions of codependence, we have come to know these behaviors as some of the ways we describe codependence. And they are. But here I am dropping out the word *codependence* and simply inviting us once again to look at specific related behaviors in a dynamic way. Seeing behaviors in this active way, on a continuum, will continue to be our theme as this book progresses.

Looking at the continuum itself, we see that on one end of the line is written "OK" and at the other end is "Going Too Far." Again, these words and their meanings are straightforward, and I will say a bit more about each end.

The "OK" end is there to acknowledge the reality that any of these giving/fixing/caretaking behaviors can be just fine depending on the situation. One of the reasons the meaning of codependence has suffered is because people have come to think and even joke that any helping or caring would be codependent. "I would have opened the door for you, but I didn't want to be codependent." "She is such a codependent. She takes her kids to school every day."

Lots of giving/fixing/caretaking is not only acceptable, but it is desirable, appropriate, and human. To offer our self to another person can be a lovely and meaningful experience for both of us.

The problems come when our offering of our self is no longer mutually beneficial. That can be visualized by traveling down this continuum and coming into the zone of "Going Too Far."

"Going Too Far" means that our giving of our self to someone else is now having a cost to each of us, a cost that can range from noticeable to gigantic.

First let's look at the cost to the other person. One way to think of codependence is to consider it as doing for someone else what he or she could do for his or her self. When we do for others what they could do on their own, we are keeping them from their own learning and growing. We could compare it in some ways to a muscle that atrophies from disuse. By unnecessarily doing for others, we are inviting atrophy of their brain and talents. Granted, we are probably not trying to cause this atrophy, but our overperforming and overdoing can certainly have this effect.

Other costs to others of our "going too far" may include offending them, hurting their feelings, and/or disempowering them.

Our actions may cause them to feel and/or believe that they are ill-equipped for the task at hand or unable to meet our expectations. This disempowering can be powerful psychologically. When a person feels helpless, they can develop hopelessness and other related symptoms of depression. I am sure most of us do not want our helping to hurt the other person in any of these ways, but it is important to remember this as we take things out of the hands of others and put them into our own hands—both literally and figuratively.

And "going too far" to extend our self can be obnoxious and just too much. It can get on the others' nerves and even make them angry, depending on how many times they have said no thanks or how many ways they have declined our offers or even started to avoid us because we are just too much. In such cases, we are moving way down the line of this continuum into the zone of "Going Too Far," and would do well to note that. Such noting can serve us well, minimizing costs to others as well as to our self. And what might those costs of "going too far" be to self?

When we overextend our self we may become fatigued, exhausted, and/or physically ill. We may become irritable, mad, disappointed, frustrated, discouraged, and/or unhappy. We are setting our self up for disappointment. We believe our behaviors, whatever the cost to us, will produce the outcome we desire or think is best. When that outcome is not what happens, and we have given it our all and more, we are headed for both emotional and physical consequences that can batter our very being. As we head this way down the continuum, we may pass through a range where our giving/fixing/caretaking produces good feelings in us, such as joy, inspiration, or hope, but as we travel further and give without due respect for self and others, we can find our self in this far end of negative consequences and personal costs.

Let's look at the specific behavioral examples listed under this continuum. These are not the only behaviors that could have been placed here, nor are they necessarily the most important. They are simply easy behaviors to identify and describe as we look at giving/fixing/caretaking. The main body of this book will present a number of other behaviors to be examined in this same way of a continuum. A look at the table of contents will show you the list of those twelve behaviors to be studied.

The first behavioral description is about *making offers*. On the continuum, this behavior ranges from *making offers within your resources* (e.g., money, time, energy) to *making offers outside of your resources* and, perhaps, carrying them out (causing debt, exhaustion, losses). On a basic level, this means to not offer money you do not have to share, to not give your time when you are overscheduled already, to not use your energy when you know it is depleted and you know you need to rest before you can really be of any help or use.

A common example I am finding with this offering behavior is in working with parents of dependent adult children. These dependent adult children are in their adulthood agewise, but for various reasons they have returned to their parent or parents' home to live. Often mental illness and/or substance abuse is part of the reason for their being dependent, but not always. The main picture is that the dependent adult child cannot support him- or herself and may not be doing much to change his or her situation. The parents are left to figure out how much to offer and when to stop offering.

These parents of dependent adult children, for example, have to figure out what offer of money is within their resources. If they decide to let their adult child have their inheritance now to live on, that may be offering within their limits. When they start giving additional money that is reducing the inheritance of the dependent adult's siblings or money that the parents may need for themselves as they age, then the givers are moving down the continuum into the zone of "Going Too Far." Many family members are being hurt by this overgiving. The dependent adult child feels no responsibility for trying to find a way to increase his or her own income. Obviously the siblings or other beneficiaries are losing and most likely will be resentful. And the parents extending their offerings down the continuum are likely increasing their own liabilities, frustrations, and resentments.

Even in the daily lives of most of us, we have rich examples of needing to pay attention to how much we are offering and how it is affecting us.

When we volunteer to be on another committee and have sworn we would not do that to our self, we are moving our self down the continuum toward "Going Too Far."

When we offer to hold the office party at our house the same week the kitchen remodeling is being completed, we are likely "going too far" in the use of many of our personal resources, including time and energy.

When we offer to keep all the children in our child's play group the day after we worked a double shift, we would do well to notice where we are placing our self on this continuum.

Because I am often working with people who offer too much, I have come to frequently suggest, "Don't offer anything that hasn't been asked for." That may sound selfish and withholding, but for those of us who are prone to giving, fixing, and caretaking, this message to our self can be very helpful in keeping us in the zone of "OK" when it comes to our giving. I know it is a useful strategy for my self.

The next behavior listed under the continuum is an extension of what we may do with our offers to someone else. That behavior is *accepting the other person's response to our offer*. On one end of the continuum is our *acceptance of the other person's acceptance or rejection of our offer.* At the other end of the continuum is our *forcing our offer on the other person.*

Forcing is rarely a good idea. I learned this especially through my twelve-step program, which teaches us that forcing can cause us problems with our thoughts and our feelings, and certainly with our relationships with others. Forcing is definitely moving down the continuum from the initial offer to insisting we know what is best and giving it to the person even though they have said no thanks.

We may think we know what is best for others, but that is for them to decide. When we do this forcing we are certainly damaging ourselves and others in the interaction. It puts others on the spot to receive what they said they did not want. They have to figure out what they want to do with what we are giving them, and I imagine they are full of mixed feelings, including awkwardness and perhaps anger. We have put our self in an equally awkward spot, because the giving we are so intent on doing may not be received as joyfully and gratefully as we would have expected. Then we may become angry as well.

Yes, this giving is likely coming from a good place in our hearts, but here we are studying codependence and the ways our generous giving can cause us problems.

Let's look again at the example of parents of dependent adult children. These parents may well start by offering within their own limits. Let's use money as an example here. "We can only afford to give you $200 per month toward your expenses." Then, as they see the reality of their child not having enough money to fix his or her car or see a doctor, they may start moving down the continuum toward giving more money, even if their child has said, "Please don't." The parents may be confronting their own guilt as they try to keep their offers within their limits. They also may be encountering all sorts of rationalizations, including "We can't take the money with us," or "This will be the last time we do this."

No, we can't take our money with us, but believe it or not, giving it away without consideration of its effects on everyone involved in the interaction can lead to problems. Not honoring someone else's "no" or our own "no" can definitely lead to bad thoughts and feelings.

What are other common ways this forcing may occur?

We have offered to bring dinner to a friend who is recovering from surgery. She has graciously declined, saying she is going to bed early and has plenty of food. We show up anyway with dinner. The house is dark as we ring the bell. She comes to the door half-asleep.

Our child in college has overdrawn his checking account. We offer to fix this situation. He says no, wanting to remedy the problem himself. We go ahead and put money in his account. When he finds this out, he calls us and is mad, because he thinks we don't have trust in his ability to take care of his own problems.

We offer to show our friend how to change the oil in her car. She is eager to learn this to be self-sufficient and save money. We change the oil for her, never showing her how to do it for herself.

The examples could go on and on. If we are not careful in our helping, we are traveling down that continuum from offers to help, teach, or serve to doing for others what they could do for themselves. We are taking their decisions, desires, and tools out of their hands and doing it for them or even despite them.

The third behavioral example under the continuum is yet another variation on this theme of offering and forcing. In this example the behavior is *making suggestions* to someone versus *insisting* that those suggestions happen. Specifically, at the "OK" end of the continuum it states that we can *make suggestions and then leave them alone*. At the "Going Too Far" end of the continuum, we *insist upon our suggestions or actually carry them out for the other person*.

I have done that—carried out my suggestion offered to someone else. Let's say I was excited about a job possibility I came upon that I thought would be perfect for someone I knew needed a job. I told him about the job. I told him about the job again. He gave no real response, so I decided he needed more information from me so he could act on this great opportunity, as I saw it. I went on the Internet and found more contact information. I told him about it, and he did nothing. So I went ahead and called to ask more details about the job. At that point, the person to whom I was offering this suggestion got angry with me and the entire effort ended.

If we are offering suggestions to our young children, that is one thing, because they are still dependent on us. In fact, even if we are offering suggestions to our children, but the suggestions are really something we know they need to do, we should be direct and not imply that what is suggested is optional.

But in this book I am usually talking about two adults learning to relate to each other in respectful, healthy ways. So when one adult makes a suggestion to the other, and it is truly a suggestion, then best to offer and leave it with the other person. The idea or information is now his or hers.

Returning to the example of the parents of the dependent adult child, let's say that the parents have learned of a financially reasonable housing situation that they believe their dependent adult child would like and could afford. Now remember, if they mean this as a requirement rather than a suggestion, they should say so right from the start and act accordingly. But let's say, for the sake of our example here, that they mean it only as a suggestion. They tell their dependent adult child about the opportunity. The dependent adult child does nothing in response. The parents decide to call and arrange a visit for all of them to go see this living space. They tell their child about this appointment. The parents show up to see the space and their dependent adult child does not come. The parents are furious. The dependent adult child says nothing.

Clearly this has become a tangled relationship. The parents are very invested in helping their dependent adult child find a place to live. In fact, they are way more invested than the child is invested. It is not clear if the child is interested at all. This may be almost totally the agenda of the parents. They were trying to help but have now moved down the continuum to a place where they are bothered and probably feel like they don't know what to do. Their helping is now hurting them, at least, and likely hurting their dependent adult child, though the child's expression of those feelings is passive and thus hard to know. Let's assume, though, that damage is being done to the child as well.

I will carry this example a bit further, since I can imagine the reader is wondering, "So what *can* the parents do?" I will take us back a couple of paragraphs and say that in this tangled time, the parents will have to decide if they really do mean that their child has to move out of their house. If they do mean that, then they will have to state that and have ways to enforce it. That's its own work for the parents. If this truly was a suggestion, then they will have to remind themselves of that and move back down the continuum, remembering that they were the ones who wanted to see this possible living place, and their child never expressed any interest in it.

In other words, as we work with our self in this way, noticing our placement on this continuum, we have to stop and assess what we really mean, and try to convey that to the other person. We have to know if it is a suggestion or a requirement. We have to notice if we are the ones who are interested and excited, and we have to remember we can't make that other person feel the same way that we may feel. We have to assess our investment in our suggestion and work to understand why we are so invested in it. Our understanding of our investment will help us greatly to know how far and in what way we should be pressing the issue.

To round out these examples of *making suggestions,* here are some other possible common examples.

We suggest to a friend that she might want to use the dog trainer we have used. She declines our suggestion, saying she has found her own. We contact our trainer anyway and have our trainer call our friend as a possible new referral.

Our child has a school project. He has asked us to get a piece of white poster board for him. We suggest that yellow would look better for what he is doing. He declines the suggestion and asks again for white. We show up at home with a piece of yellow poster board for him.

We are visiting our mother-in-law and notice that her spices are randomly located in her kitchen. We suggest that if they were in one place and organized, they would be so much easier to use. She shrugs and walks out of the room. While she is out of the house, we arrange her spices as we suggested.

The examples are powerful and speak for themselves. Yes, with very little noticing on our part we can move our self from an offer to a forcing, from a suggestion to an insistence. Most often we mean well as we start, but the situation and our self deteriorate as we move into that zone of "Going Too Far."

That is our mission here: to learn to notice our behaviors, our investments in our offers, the reasons for our investments, and the progression of our behaviors and emotional states as we move from "OK" to "Going Too Far."

Most importantly, our mission is to learn to modulate our self so that what was good and fine as we started does not become soured.

This practical story of codependence offers visual ways to consider the dynamics of codependence. Looking at our behaviors as we interact with others, it can be useful to remember **the balance scale, the circles, and the continuum.** Each may have an appeal to particular individuals, and each can have a particular usefulness depending on the situation to which we are paying attention.

The continuum is the visual tool we will continue to use within this book. In fact, the continuum is the basis of how we will study the forthcoming lessons from the border collie and me. I consider the continuum to be a useful way to differentiate between healthy and unhealthy behaviors. It can help us to detect where we may be shifting from helping to hurting, from offering to controlling, from fixing to breaking.

Let's see what I mean.

With these various ways of understanding codependence in place—personal, professional, and practical—it's time to get to the Tales and Lessons.

*T*he issue seemed to be that he had never seen mailboxes on posts; there was no way he was going to go near them. I reviewed the list of border collie characteristics in my mind. No one had included the word neurotic, and I was starting to panic.[1]

* * *

I watched all of the border collie behaviors for a short time and decided that the only way for this dog to have a good life was to provide him with training and a fairly intensive schedule of activities.[2]

—Mary Burch

preamble

D aisy stares at me on a regular basis these days, saying to me, I am sure, "Work on our book!" I know that is a message I am giving my self, and I choose to believe she is saying the same thing, since we are kindred spirits, you know.

As I write, Daisy often lies on the floor nearby, looking up occasionally and following me to the kitchen or bathroom as I take my short breaks. She is now sixteen years old and still is in very good health. She has herded me to this work and does a good job of helping to hold me in place and keep me company.

This book was to be a simple book, written primarily out of my experiences in working with codependence and my experiences of living with and loving my border collie, Daisy. As I have worked on it, I have chosen to enrich it by adding the more detailed descriptions of codependence and reference sources, and I did some reading about border collies. That reading about border collies was rich and entertaining for me. What the author was writing about was amazingly consistent with how I have experienced Daisy and how I experience codependence. On several occasions of reading this material I said to my husband, "I could change the words *border collie* to *codependent,* and the sentence would still be accurate." Here are a few of those sentences:

"First and foremost, the border collie is a working dog. Relied upon for centuries to work at the side of shepherds, border collies have been selectively bred for intelligence and versatility . . . . This is a tireless, high energy breed requiring owners who are firmly committed to providing stimulating work activities for the dog . . . . Without meaningful work, border collies will become bored and depressed and may develop behavior problems."[3]

"The border collie is a working dog who thrives on having a job to do and a purpose in life."[4]

"Border collies are typically described as highly intelligent, very trainable, physical, adaptable, lively, athletic, fast, hardworking, loyal, tenacious, sensitive, and most important, extremely tractable."[5]

"Border collies have such an intense desire to please that they can suffer from 'fear of failure.'"[6]

For me, these descriptors echo many of the characteristics of codependence I wrote about in "The Codependency Story" in the previous section. The codependent is a hardworking person who desires to help and to fix and to please. The codependent is a person who notices the needs of others and can adapt and respond to those needs. The codependent does well with focused tasks and clear purpose.

To share my thinking further with you, let's look at the following lists. The first column is a list of border collie characteristics I derived from Mary Burch.[7] The second column lists the four core defining features of codependency identified by Dear, Roberts, and Lange[8] and Dear and Roberts.[9] The third column is a distilled list of the qualities and behaviors we will be examining as I tell the border collie Tales and Lessons. These are the behaviors I have come to see that Daisy and I share and that capture the essence of what is good and what can be troubling about codependence.

Border Collie Characteristics	Defining Features of Codependency	Tales and Lessons
Highly intelligent	External focusing	Smart
Alert	Self-sacrificing	Devoted
Responsive	Interpersonal control	Hardworking
Hardworking	Emotional suppression	Serving
Athletic		People pleasing
Loyal		Sensitive
Tenacious		Adaptable
Sensitive		Herding
Very active		Reactive
Affectionate		Tenacious
Eager to learn		Delighted
Eager to please		Big-hearted
Thrives on human companionship		

I am pleased with these lists. Though they read simply, they are the result of much thinking and research. Again, as I started writing this book, I was creating it from an honest and yet whimsical spirit. Having lived with Daisy and been in recovery for my own codependence, I could see the similarities between us, and those similarities both amused me and educated me. I thought I would write essays that would convey both this amusement and my education.

Then, as the years have passed and I have only been able to work on this book sporadically, I have studied, learned, and taught more on this topic of codependence. And I have been blessed with Daisy having good health and a long life over these same years, thus adding to my collection of experiences. So the book has evolved, adding more meaning to whimsy. It always was to be meaningful, and by sharing with you some of the literature sources of what I am writing, I trust you can gain an even deeper understanding of this topic and of your self.

Looking at the three lists, I see them almost as a formula for the characteristics we will be examining in the Tales and Lessons. The first two columns add together to create the third column, those characteristics Daisy and I share.

As we move into the Tales and Lessons, I will be using a particular format for each chapter. I will first present a section entitled "Characteristic Described," in which I offer both definitions and behavioral descriptions of the characteristic studied in that chapter— a characteristic known to be true of the border collie, the codependent, and me. It is in this section that I want to help you to see how a particular characteristic or trait or quality can be expressed through active behaviors, as I discussed earlier. It is by noticing our behaviors that we are able to make constructive changes for our self. We can describe a person as being nice. It is hard for a person to change their niceness, even if he or she wants to do so, without understanding the behaviors he or she exhibits that reflect niceness: offering help, giving ideas, complimenting, and doing things for others. Each chapter will look at a particular characteristic shared by the border collie and the codependent and talk about that characteristic in terms of active behaviors we can learn to notice and moderate.

We then will move into the "Tales Told" of Daisy and me.

Finally, the "Lessons Learned" in each chapter will again highlight the importance of seeing these lessons in terms of behaviors on a continuum. Each of these characteristics in the Tales and Lessons can be wonderful, and each can be problematic. Our overall lesson is to learn where we are starting to go too far with that particular behavior and then what to do with our self.

I am not the only writer on codependence who thinks of these behaviors on a continuum. Gary Fisher and Thomas Harrison explain that codependent characteristics are not necessarily good or bad. Sometimes those characteristics are adaptive, useful, and satisfying. At other times those same characteristics are problematic. They suggest that we see codependence as a cluster of behaviors on a continuum ranging from mild to severe, and determine where an individual falls on the continuum by noting the extent to which the individual's emotions and functioning are affected by his or her codependent behaviors.[10]

In a more recent text on treating codependence, Zelvin also supports this viewing of codependence on a continuum ranging from mild to severe. She suggests the use of the continuum as a way to make the broad application of the word *codependence* more meaningful and useful.[11]

As early as 1990, in writing about codependence in her resource book, Yoder speaks of codependence as progressing in the same ways as addiction. With codependence, she maintains, people lose control over their own thoughts and feelings and behaviors as they become preoccupied with other people. To illustrate this progression of codependence, Yoder offers some clear behavioral descriptors of this process: helping can become taking responsibility for the lives of others; compassion can become taking on the identity of others; sharing knowledge and ideas can become taking over the lives of others, while the codependent's own life disappears.[12]

This progression that Yoder describes is similar to the approach I use with each of the behaviors described in Tales and Lessons. On one end of the continuum we will examine the behavior itself, understanding its meaning and primarily seeing its value and strengths. As we look at its progression down the continuum, however, we will see how that very behavior can become too much for us and others. We will see how we *can* lose control over our self—how, in fact, we *can* lose control over our thoughts, feelings, and actions, and thus how what began as not a problem is now a problem.

You can call this an addiction or not. In the ways we do lose control over our self, I agree that it is acting like an addictive process. Loss of control over whatever the substance or process may be is a fundamental way I diagnose addiction. For our work here in this book, however, my primary intent is not to argue the point of whether codependence is or is not a relationship addiction. My work here is primarily functional, inviting you to simply look at the behaviors that we describe as codependent and to see how they can work for you, at what point they become problematic, and what to do to moderate those behaviors and not lose your self.

I'm ready for some Tales and Lessons.

I imagine you are, too.

Smart

*"I can learn
new tricks."*

Characteristic Described

I am starting with "Smart" intentionally. I think it is important to understand that codependence does not have anything to do with how smart a person is. Many codependents are very smart.

So what do I mean by smart? Smartness involves a number of abilities including learning new material, learning from experience, problem solving, imagining what we cannot see, and being able to generalize from one learning to others. It also involves having a good memory, language, and vocabulary; self-awareness; awareness of others; logical reasoning; abstract reasoning; flexibility; and creativity.

These mental abilities are most commonly attributed to humans as a hallmark of what differentiates us from animals; however, research studies are showing us that these advanced abilities can be found in other species as well. In March 2008, *National Geographic* took a look at this research in an article titled "Minds of Their Own: Animals Are Smarter than You Think."[13] Among the animals they wrote about was the border collie.

In this article, Virginia Morell reports on two border collies with large vocabularies. Rico, who appeared on television in Germany in 2001, knew at least 200 words and was able to learn new words as quickly as a toddler. And Betsy had a vocabulary of 300 words.

Juliane Kaminski, a cognitive psychologist studying both Rico and Betsy, suggests that the border collie is good at communication because it is a motivated working dog that has to listen closely to its owner in order to perform its tasks and complete its work.

Supporting this understanding of the border collie's intelligence, Mary Burch has many things to say. "Border collies must be intelligent and responsive to training in order to perform the jobs for which they were bred . . . . A border collie's eagerness to learn and to please enables the dog to be trained to perform complex tasks." [14]

She further explains that their intelligence is needed as they herd and problem solve, sometimes at long distances from their handlers. "Border collies are typically described as highly intelligent, very trainable . . . adaptable . . . and, most important, extremely tractable." [15]

I had to look up "tractable." I wasn't really sure of its meaning. *Merriam-Webster's Collegiate Dictionary* defines "tractable" as 1) capable of being easily led, taught, or controlled; 2) easily handled, managed, or wrought.*

I was impressed. This definition of *tractable* can so apply to the strengths and weaknesses of codependent behavior.

The strengths of smartness and our ability to learn are clear and extremely desirable. We want to be able to learn, problem solve, expand our understanding of things, be able to think on our own, and be able to apply what we are learning. We want to be able to think clearly and trust our own intelligence.

*By permission. From *Merriam-Webster's Collegiate® Dictionary*, 11th Edition ©2012 by Merriam-Webster, Incorporated (www.Merriam-Webster.com).

The weakness comes in when we are unable to fully use our intelligence. What in the world would cause us to do that? Well, a number of things.

First of all, we may not be aware of and/or willing to use our intelligence. Perhaps you have had experiences that left you feeling not very smart. Perhaps other people told you that you are not very smart. These experiences certainly distance us from our intelligence and decrease the chances that we will use it. Or perhaps you've had successful experiences that indicated you are smart, but you are unwilling to trust your self and use those abilities. You downplay your ability to think and learn. You deny it or ignore it.

We also are not fully using our intelligence or common sense when we are operating out of a programmed self. This programmed self is where codependent behaviors can become a problem. The definitions of *tractable* presented above include features of being easily led or controlled, easily managed. In our efforts to live with our self and others, we do not want to allow our intelligence to be reduced to trained behaviors and thoughts. It is good that we can be trained; that's part of what's called learning. But we do not want to allow that training to always dictate our behaviors. We want to be able to learn and then use our intelligence to know if and when we should apply what we have learned.

These considerations are so relevant to several of the defining features of codependency.[16] These core elements that are coming to light as we look at intelligence include *external focusing, self-sacrificing,* and *emotional suppression.*

External focusing, or focusing outside of our self, can mean that we pay so much attention to the thoughts, needs, emotions, and behaviors of others that we do not pay attention to our own, or we modify our self to accommodate what we see and believe about people and things outside of our self. Often this type of external focus is necessary for initial learning, but we do not need to allow our learning to remain exclusively external. We need to incorporate it with our internal.

Expanding on this point about the need for both external and internal as we learn, it is useful to be aware of *self-sacrificing*, which can involve responding to others to the neglect of self. It is important to learn both the needs of others and our self. Then, it is equally important to be able to not respond to others in an automatic, programmed way that can ignore our own needs, but rather respond in a thoughtful way that uses our intelligence by considering the multiple variables involved and then making a decision about how to respond.

Additionally, our ability to use our intelligence can be drastically affected by our emotions. The presence of strong emotional states can overpower our ability to think and use what we have already learned. When we do psychological testing, we are asked to assess whether we think the person's performance on the tests is accurate to his or her abilities. One of the important things for us to consider with that question is the emotional condition of the person during the testing. If the person was calm and rested, the results are probably more accurate than if he or she was fearful, anxious, resistant, or any of a number of other powerful emotions, including feelings of love.

It is important for us to be aware of our emotions and to be able to manage them so we can use the intelligence we do have. *Emotional suppression* means that we are not letting our emotions into our awareness. When we do this, there is the likelihood that they will overwhelm us and be expressed in indirect and/or damaging ways. And who can think under such circumstances?

Daisy was once the Reserve Grand Champion at the Rockbridge Regional Fair. That was a fine moment, but also, not really that big. The Rockbridge Regional Fair is a wonderful event held in our county near Lexington, Virginia. As the name says, it is a regional fair full of rides and 4-H demonstrations and competitions.

Prior to the fair, my daughter Grace and her best friend Amy had taken their dogs to a series of 4-H dog training classes at a local barn. Daisy had already gone to dog obedience classes with Monty when she first came to us, so she had some basics. The 4-H class reiterated those lessons and gave Daisy another opportunity to practice these skills in the company of other dogs. To tell the truth, Grace and Amy, along with their dogs, Daisy and Zeus, were the only students who seemed to be taking the classes with some seriousness and intent. In fact, sometimes they were the only ones in the class.

So when it came time for the competition at the fair, Daisy and Zeus had some advantages. In a big arena with a dirt floor, all of the dogs and their owners made a large circle, with each owner controlling his or her dog on a leash and demonstrating commands as they were given. Daisy did beautifully with her commands, but in between them, Grace had to work with her to get her to stay in place and calm down. She was so excited, seemingly with joy, and brimming with energy that Grace quietly had to repeatedly tell her to "sit" and "stay." And she would.

Zeus, on the other hand, not only knew and executed his commands, but also was a much cooler and calmer competitor. So when it came time for the awards, Zeus was named the Grand Champion of the Rockbridge Regional Fair, and, as you know, Daisy was named the Reserve Grand Champion.

Yes, Daisy is plenty smart. She knows many words and commands, though probably not nearly 300. We talk to Daisy all the time, so she knows not only the basics, including her name, "sit," "stay," "down," and "stop," but also phrases such as "stay by me" and "stay in the yard." We have to spell words such as "walk" and "creek" and "river" so that we don't unnecessarily excite Daisy about such outings if we are only discussing their possibility.

And yes, Daisy can be trained to do new things, especially if a treat is involved. Daisy's first dog training classes involved the use of small food bites, and I have continued this practice with her. Treats are given for good behavior, with or without human prompting. Several years ago my stepdaughter Ava was visiting us from Houston, where she lives. Hanging out in our kitchen, she was watching Daisy respond to the prospect of a reward and said, "It's amazing what that word *treat* can do for her." The knowledge of getting her treat can help Daisy to calm her excited, active self or stop something she really wants to do and come to me. These are things she has learned. I know Daisy is paying attention to this world in which she lives and is using her brain to calculate what is expected of her and how she wants to respond to get what she wants.

But Daisy sometimes has her limits in using her smartness. She is not 100 percent responsive to commands. If we are on a walk and she is following some really good scent, she is reluctant to "come," and we worry that she could get lost or run out into a road because she is not thinking about what she is doing. If Daisy has taken to barking at nothing that we can see or hear and we try to quiet her by calm reassurance or a simple command of "quiet," she may persist despite reasonable efforts to teach her otherwise.

*   *   *   *   *

I was wondering how I was going to transition from Daisy's tale of smartness to mine, and the very sentences of this last paragraph have set me up well.

"If she is following some really good scent . . . she could get lost or run out into a road." The phrase "following some really good scent" is striking to me. I am sure I have had my attention drawn to some really good "scent" and subsequently lost my self in it and nearly "run out into a road." The "scent" could be a person, an idea, a plan, an inspiration. And the phrase "she may persist despite reasonable efforts to teach her otherwise" speaks as well to my own persistence that wants to defy the facts and reality of the person and/or situation that has my attention.

The easiest tale for me to tell about my self here is about my earlier years in my relationship with my husband. Much of that tale is told in detail in the earlier section of this book, "The Codependency Story: Personal." Here I will tell one particular tale illustrating, among many things, smartness.

Like Daisy, I have a few titles that speak to my smartness. I was the valedictorian of my high school graduation class. I attended a prestigious college. I have several professional licenses and certificates. I have written a published book. I have a good brain and am very grateful for it. I can learn and process and create. And I can work my self into an emotional state that limits my use of those abilities.

Relationships can really bring this out in us. At least I know that is true for me. When I first met my husband, I was taken by him right from the start. I wasn't hungry for a relationship at that time. In fact, I was seeing someone else on a regular basis and had a few other invites waiting to happen. But when I met Monty, my brain started to suffer some interference. It happened to me gradually but noticeably.

What started to come up for me was insecurity, jealousy,

fearfulness, and wishing I looked a different way or thought a different way or was just plain someone else. I started to believe that who I am was not okay or enough. Almost all of these emotions were my creations. They did not have anything to do with things Monty said to me or things he did. Yes, I have said that in those earlier years Monty was an active alcoholic, but he did not have several girlfriends at the same time he was seeing me, nor did he criticize my appearance or ways. I just became so attached to wanting him to like me (the "scent") that I wasn't thinking straight. I would notice what he seemed to like and would try to be that way. He did not, for the most part, know that all of this was going on inside me. He only knew through my occasional meltdowns or emotional outbursts that something was wrong with me.

I remember being in a restaurant with Monty and a good friend of his in Baltimore, Maryland, many years ago. The restaurant was full and lively, and we were glad to get a table in one of the rooms. Monty and I were sitting on one side of the table, with his friend on the other side. We were enjoying ourselves and trying to hear one another over the sounds of the room. I noticed several tables down from us a group of women our age having a fun time talking and laughing. I decided that one of them facing our way was particularly attractive and appealing in her energy and style. I started to watch her and watch Monty out of the corner of my eye to see if he was noticing her. I decided he was. So I watched some more.

As I watched, I got sicker and sicker. I was trying to act normal but was losing my appetite and general interest in dinner. And my thinking really started to deteriorate. I wished I was like this woman, this complete stranger to us all. I wished I was attractive like her. I wished I was so engaging and such good company. I wished I could be such fun to be with. I watched and watched and started to believe that at any point Monty could get up from our table and go join her, leaving me. I really thought that was a possibility.

I contained all of this emotion and crazy thinking until we left the restaurant. I do not remember who left first, our group or theirs, but I do know that I had some big meltdown with Monty when we got back to his friend's house. I told him how scared I was that he was going to leave me, that I was not who he wanted to be with, that I was not fun and exciting. I asked him about the woman I had been watching in the restaurant and compared my self to her. I accused him of being interested in her and asked why he didn't just go and join her since he was so interested!

Monty hardly knew what I was talking about. He said he had noticed that group of women, as they were clearly having a good time, but there was no more to it for him than that. He really didn't know what to say to me. Here I was, so worked up about all that I had been telling my self about me, him, and "the other woman," and he was just having dinner in a restaurant.

I had created my own reality with that situation. I had abandoned my good thinking and created a story of my own. My emotions took over along with some of my own inaccurate notions about my self and my abilities and qualities. Once these emotions and thoughts took hold, I spiraled downward as they escalated to the top and took control. Who would have believed that the valedictorian of her high school class could function this way? Who would have believed that a graduate of the College of William & Mary would think in such a crazy way and act in such a needy and undignified manner?

Well, I'm here to admit that such craziness is possible even among the smart. Smart is good but has its limits if it is not coupled with reality, emotional centeredness, and common sense. My dad would say to me, "Petey, you have a good brain, but sometimes I wonder about why you don't use your common sense, too."

I'm learning.

Lessons Learned

In applying "smart" to the continuum model, I put the healthy use of our smartness in the middle of the line, at the point of balance. Each end of this continuum, or balance scale, represents distortions of our smartness: at the left end distortions by emotions, and at the right end distortions by overintellectualizing. Looking at this in more detail, at the left end of the continuum I see smartness with interference from emotions as well as mistakes we are making in our thinking—thoughts we are holding onto that are not accurate and that are negatively affecting our emotions. Both our emotional state and errors in our thinking can substantially diminish the benefits of our smartness. At the right end of the continuum I put smartness without use of good common sense, smartness gone wild in analyzing and overanalyzing itself—trying to use brains to figure out, unsuccessfully, something that would be helped more by good judgment based on the present reality and/or the accessing of intuition and spirituality.

I can range all over this continuum. I can be so upset that I can't think straight. I can make emotional decisions that I will likely later regret. I can also get caught up in my thinking, trying to figure out what this or that means *ad nauseam,* and trying to problem solve or come to some conclusion that I want to be true rather than seeing the present facts and living with them for the time being. Just like Daisy, I can know what I have learned and still ignore it and go after what I want in that moment—and for both of us, that can be a dangerous thing to do.

I have learned:

It is important for me to honor my smartness. I have been blessed with a good brain and ability to think. So have you, whatever you have been told and whatever you believe about your ability. Being smart involves both native abilities and our cultivation of those abilities.

It is important for me to connect with my intelligence in a healthy way, recognizing it, doing things to develop it, and using it often.

I can develop my smartness. As a child, teenager, and young adult, I was always a good student. School appealed to me. I liked assignments and doing them well. I am sure those activities helped to develop my intelligence. Just as we took Daisy to dog obedience classes to learn and use her abilities, school did the same thing for me. Now, as an adult, I want to keep using my brain. You can, too, whether you did much with school or not. We can read and write and take classes. We can work puzzles and learn new skills and crafts. We can work out with our body in ways that makes our brains work, such as learning dance steps or playing a sport or game that involves strategy.

I want to be able to think. Developing my intelligence certainly can enable me to think better. It strengthens those brain muscles and gives me something to use. I have found that if I am not careful, I can fall into automatic, habitual behaviors and not think much at all. Someone can ask me what I think of something, and I realize I have given it no thought. I can do things "because we have always done them that way," and not give a thought to being creative or just plain practical about whatever it is that I am doing.

I want to be able to think for my self. I want to not only be able to think as thinking applies to daily life, to problem solving, and to planning, but also to use thinking for my very self. I want to know what I think about particular people, places, and things. I want to have my opinions and ideas. I don't want to just say, "Whatever you want." Years ago a client of mine was actively working on learning to do this thinking for her self. She was pleased to be doing so. In one session, she reported that she had shared some ideas of her own with her husband. Not used to hearing such things from her, he disapprovingly asked, "Who's been putting those thoughts into your head?" We don't want to be full of thoughts put there by others. I guess her husband could not imagine that she was able to think for herself, and quite frankly, I do not believe that he wanted her to do so. If anyone was going to put thoughts into her head, he believed, it should be him. Our health depends on us learning to think for our self: What is it I want? What is it I need in this moment or for this day? Think, Nancy, think. Use your brain to attend to you.

I must be aware of and manage my emotions in order to be able to think for my self. Anxiety, in particular, is an emotion that can cripple my thinking. Anger can, too, as well as love. If I am aware, I can feel the increased adrenaline in my body in those situations of heightened emotion. I can see my preoccupations with the identified source of my feelings and watch as my ability to think and use my brain diminishes. Just yesterday I was in a situation that raised my anxiety tremendously. Part of the anxiety came from having to wait in the unknown about a potentially dangerous situation. During that waiting time, when I had done all I could do, I tried to get other things done that involved my brain, such as bookkeeping and banking. It was so interesting to observe how many mistakes I made in doing these common tasks. I was using liquid paper to correct errors and started to triple-check my work in light of my obvious handicaps caused by my anxiety. I brought my awareness of my emotions into play rather than allowing my self to be totally lost in them.

I can manage powerful emotions by noticing the thoughts I am having connected with those emotions. Usually those thoughts are extreme or disastrous. I am predicting abandonment, rejection, loss, death. If I am not aware and ready to work, those inaccurate thoughts will dominate, and my ability to use my more rational, balanced thinking will be gone. Cognitive-behavioral psychology is about learning to notice the errors in our thinking and correcting them. This can be a tough exercise, because we can become attached so quickly to our beliefs, which can become our obstacle to using our brain. I must notice the thought(s) feeding my emotional state (e.g., *Something very bad has happened that is keeping him from answering his phone*) and develop an alternative thought that is more accurate and balanced (e.g., *For some reason he is not answering his phone. I have no reason to expect that harm has occurred. I will leave a message and trust I will hear from him as soon as that is possible.*).

I can help manage my emotions by mindfully being in the present moment. Once I have brought my awareness to my emotional state, I can help my self further by not only correcting my thoughts, but also by quieting my thoughts. This, too, can be a big challenge. Sometimes when I suggest this idea to others, they cannot imagine this being possible. Well, it is. Mindfulness can be a very useful path to this goal. You will hear me speak of mindfulness often in this book as a way to help balance our codependent behaviors. Jon Kabat-Zinn's book *Full Catastrophe Living* is an original text for what I am making quick reference to here.[17] Mindfulness means that we train our self to come back over and over to the present moment by allowing our focus to be on our natural breath and/or present bodily senses and sensations. To do this requires intentional practice. And it is worth it in terms of developing a healthier relationship with our emotions and thoughts so they won't run away with us.

With quieter emotions and thoughts, I am better able to access my brain. I can be more rational. I am likely to still be carrying the feelings and thoughts that were so disturbing to me, but now they are not dominating. Unlike Daisy, I am not persisting in my barking "despite reasonable efforts to teach me otherwise." I can quiet and calm my self, sit better with what is, and use my brain as I choose.

I don't want to overuse my brain. This speaks to the other end of our "Smart" continuum where we can overthink and overanalyze. When we are thinking constantly about particular things, we call this ruminating. We go over and over the same thoughts, whether we are awake or asleep. We try to imagine all possible scenarios (which we can't) and imagine all types of solutions (which we can't). This is where we are not using our smartness to its best advantage. I try to notice when I am doing this and stop it using the same cognitive corrections and mindfulness I described above. "Give it a break," I say to my self as my thoughts spin on.

By giving a break to my persistent thoughts, I can access my common sense and intuition, both of which make me smarter. I know that there is enormous value in both.

My common sense can offer great practicality and reasonableness. Whether my common sense is blocked by emotionality or overanalyzing, I am not as smart as I can be if I cannot use it. It is my common sense that may help me to see that a particular person, place, or thing is not good for me. It is my common sense that can help me to protect and care for my self better. I *can* "learn new tricks," but do I want to? Are they good for me? Are they *my* new tricks that will advance me, or is someone else teaching me tricks that will lead me into a relationship or situation that is not good for me? It is good to learn, and it is important to add common sense. Over the years of being a therapist I have come to see that one of the major things I offer to clients is often a commonsense observation or a statement about the obvious relative to their situation. It can be very freeing to simply realize the obvious: "Oh, I really don't have time to do that." "No, that job isn't good for me." "I shouldn't call him back." Common sense is a good idea, and I am much smarter when I am using it.

I can be brilliant when I use my intuition. Some of my best thoughts and ideas have come from not thinking, from quieting my self and noticing what emerges. In many ways that is how I write. If I get too much into thinking about words and concepts, I block my ability to let them flow out onto the paper. Intuition and spirit mingle together for me. They involve listening, being open, and noticing. When I can work in this way, all sorts of other thoughts, ideas, and feelings come forward, and the potential for brilliance is there. I cannot make this happen; I just have to know that this type of smartness is possible and just allow my self to be. I continue to be a student of this process, and I haven't yet been able to teach Daisy how to do this. Imagine how smart we both could become.

devoted

....

*"All I want to do
is watch you."*

Characteristic Described

My idea for this book started from my noticing Daisy's devotion to me, devotion expressed particularly by the extent to which she attends to and watches me. A tale about that is soon to come. First, let's look at devotion.

Merriam-Webster's Collegiate Dictionary defines *devotion* as "the fact or state of being ardently dedicated and loyal (as to an idea or person . . . *devote* is likely to imply compelling motives and often attachment to an objective."*

I like these strong words as we look at devotion, words such as *ardent, loyal, compelling,* and *attachment.* In a healthy way, devotion is important. It is good for us to know what we believe and to what we are committed. Loyalty is nearly imperative in a good relationship. Trust and safety flow naturally from loyalty.

And loyalty can go too far. We can allow our devotion to cloud our judgment and contribute to decision making that is harmful to us.

*By permission. From *Merriam-Webster's Collegiate® Dictionary*, 11th Edition ©2012 by Merriam-Webster, Incorporated (www.Merriam-Webster.com).

Our loyalty can cause us to disregard boundaries we have set for our self and the other person. Our loyalty can cause us to do for others what they need to be doing for themselves. We can become too ardent and too attached to the object or our devotion and lose sight of our self. While we're watching another, we're not watching our self.

In talking about the border collie, Burch always includes *loyal* as a descriptor, and she elaborates on that characteristic by looking at the dog's ability to watch and attend to the owner's moods and expressions as an extension of the animal's deep connection to its owner. Here's what she says:

> "It was critical to shepherds that border collies pay attention to small details. The dogs had to be able to respond to a whistle given from hundreds of yards away or to a hand signal that was given as a flock of sheep ran by. Out of this heritage evolved a dog who is very discriminating with regard to an owner's moods and expressions."[18]

In describing a utility-level obedience competition with her border collie, Burch illustrates this powerful attending connection:

> "Just as he turned and faced me, I thought about how we had gotten through our problem area successfully. I smiled and literally breathed a small sigh of relief. Too late to change my expression, I saw my dog's face. He had picked up on my expression that said, 'Whew, we did it.' I knew before he moved a foot he thought we were finished for the day. He happily trotted up to me with a look that said, 'Okay, let's go back to the hotel.' We were disqualified again because he had reacted to a change in the expression on my face."[19]

What a perfect story for what I speak of here! It is devotion that runs so deep that we are literally watching and discerning and making crucial decisions based on what we think we are discerning—and how wrong all of that can go.

Two of the defining features of codependency are particularly relevant here. As described previously, *external focusing* is about placing our attention on someone else's behaviors, opinions, and expectations and then trying to obtain approval and self-esteem from that other person by adjusting our behaviors and expectations to match theirs. Devoted watching can do this. Devoted watching can have us so fully engaged in taking in the other person that we are not also taking in our self and our situation. At its core, devoted watching is about approval and reassurance—reassurance that we are okay and that the other person is okay with us.

Self-sacrificing is an extension of *external focusing*. Our external focus has us taking in not only the behaviors, opinions, and expectations of others, but also their needs. It is important here to remember that these "needs" *may* be expressed by others, but more often than not, *we* have imagined/decided what their needs are, and we are acting out of that likely inaccurate knowing, as did Mary Burch's border collie in the story above. To add to the tangle, we choose to neglect our own needs so as to accommodate their needs. This is a personal setup for the "pleasing" behaviors we will later study. Devotion can have us doing this self-neglecting and accommodation of others for a number of reasons, including approval, reassurance, and esteem, as well as notions of fixing, helping, or changing someone else.

As I worked on this chapter, several longstanding popular songs about love and devotion came to my mind. A theme that emerges is not being able to live without the other person, of not being able to imagine a life without that other person, of being so devoted as to not be able to think or do. Some lyrics even convey hopelessness and complete emptiness without the other person, as well as a commitment to him or her no matter what.

Again, healthy devotion is valuable and enriching, offering us the opportunity to connect with people and experiences outside of our self. Devotion can anchor us and help us to grow. It can also stunt our growth if our devotion has us believing we have no life without another person and are not willing to let go of him or her if needed. Surely this cannot be the experience of healthy devotion.

Tales Told

Every morning the dogs and I wake together: Daisy, of course, and Eddie, the black lab mix who joined us eight years ago. Eddie also was a wandering stray who found his way to our country yard with a broken back leg and, according to our veterinarian, had had no food for three weeks. Eddie is about sixty-five pounds, so he and Daisy make a cute, companionable pair, with Daisy being about half his size.

I don't get up the first time my alarm goes off. I put the alarm across the room from my bed, so I have to get up each time it goes off and hit the snooze button. The dogs, who sleep on their own beds on the floor by my side of the bed, know my routine. They do not get up until they see that I have hit the snooze button for the last time. They know this because I click off the alarm and remain standing, putting on enough clothes to be warm and civilized.

The three of us clatter down the wooden steps, through our living room and into our kitchen. The three cats, Miss Puddin, Zoe, and Lola, are already ahead of us, waiting for their morning treats. All six of us gather, and the five of them wait until I get my coffee on. Then it is their turn, with the cats eating soft cat food and half-and-half on their pink plates first. Then Daisy and Eddie have their food delivered to their personal bowls, followed by a cat plate for each to lick and a dog bone for each. Then out the door we go to take our morning walk, with a few more treats along the way for these good dogs.

Back in the house, peace starts settling again into our animal world. Mel, our pet rat, is given his morning treats of dog food bits and his own pellet, and Miss Puddin asks to go outside for the day. Zoe finds one of her favorite spots in the house and cleans herself. Lola, the kitten, plays and runs around, sometimes inviting Zoe to join her. Eddie heads back up to his mattress. And Daisy stays with me.

It is my turn to get ready for the day, and Daisy remains with me everywhere I go:

I'm in the kitchen fixing my coffee and food. Daisy sits at the edge of the kitchen floor watching me.

I'm in the bathroom doing things at the mirror. Daisy sits in the doorway watching me.

I move through the house gathering my things for the day. Daisy sits in the center of the living room where she knows I will repeatedly pass until I am done.

Daisy's watching is very sweet. Her brown eyes are not begging. I know when she's begging. Her watching is lovingly conveying her devotion to me, her desire to be with me, to be near me, to know what I'm doing and where I am going.

My husband commonly describes me as "Daisy's person," meaning she responds to others in our home, but I am her main person. "Daisy's Nancy is home," Monty will say as Daisy stays close to me and seems to dote. She listens best to me, comes more readily to me, will lick me as long as I will allow it, and, even as I write, she is the pet who is lying here on the floor beside my chair, keeping us both in good and loving company. Daisy is totally devoted to me.

Daisy watches me until I leave the house for the day, petting her and reassuring her as I leave that I will see her in the evening.

*   *   *   *   *

Daisy's devotion is uncensored and unyielding, and I soak it up. She is a very good friend whom I love dearly. And her intense watching behavior is familiar to me. I am a watcher, too. Let's face it: I know Daisy is watching me because I am watching her.

I have been a watcher for as long as I can remember. Some of my watchfulness is about devotion—but devotion in a mixed way. Some of my devotion is the standard "I love you, and I'm loyal and dedicated to you." And some of my devotion goes beyond these parameters into watching another person to determine "Are you mad at me? Have I displeased you? Are you disapproving of me? Am I in trouble?"

When I am feeling insecure or upset and worrying about people to whom I am devoted, I have been known to

- watch their faces for information about how they are feeling and thinking;
- watch them out of windows to see what they are doing;
- ask unnecessary questions, looking for a future orientation that includes me.

What are all these unbecoming behaviors about? In part, I believe they are about devotion gone too far.

Devotion can mean that I will stand by you, that you can count on me, that I will defend you, that I will do my part to encourage our relationship. Devotion gone too far can involve me standing by you when you have betrayed me or let me down. It can involve me defending you when you have no good defense. It can involve me not doing something that would be good for me to do. Devotion gone too far can involve me doing more than my part to make this relationship work.

So again, why would I engage in these unbecoming behaviors? I am devoted to these people, *and* I am actively seeking reassurance that they are equally devoted to me, and thus won't abandon me. Yes, fears of being abandoned are indeed feeding my watchfulness. And beneath those feelings of abandonment are my fears that they will abandon me because I have done something wrong or I am not good enough.

I know that I fall into the category of wanting to be a "good girl." This has been with me all of my life. I want to do what is right. I do not like conflict. I hate to feel like I am "in trouble." I want to be on top of my game and have everything under control, including the way others feel about me.

A simple story related to devotion has occurred over and over in my adult life and involves my discomfort with conflict. Many of us have stories about devotion that involve major life decisions— devotion juxtaposed with finances or marital status or child-rearing issues. These are glaring examples of where we have to assess the extent to which we let our devotion influence the ultimate decisions we need to make for our self. Sometimes the situations in which our devotion can help or hurt us are the smaller details of life.

I do not like to argue with my husband, yet sometimes we argue. Often the argument seems to come out of the blue. Things are going along okay, and then we hit some snag in conversation or idea, and we are mad and our communication falls apart. Usually these arguments are over very small things such as furniture and schedules and work on our lovely old house.

Years ago, in my early recovery, we had an argument over the dishes. We have had many arguments over the dishes, in fact, but here I will recount just one of them.

I like to do the dishes relatively soon after a meal, and certainly before I fix the next meal. I do not like to cook on a messy counter or with a sink full of dirty dishes. Believe me, I am not obsessive about this. Ask anyone who spends time in our home. It's just a strong preference. Monty is more casual about the dishes and will let them sit. If the dishes are his to wash, I leave them alone for a good while. But then I reach a point at which I want them washed.

Such was the case one Saturday night in our home. The dishes from dinner were stacked on the counter along with many dishes that had accumulated throughout the day. We have always had an understanding in our home that one person cooks and the other washes the dishes. I had cooked; the dishes were his to do. To the best of my memory, I asked Monty if he would wash the dishes by the next morning.

He was not pleased with this request of mine. Perhaps it seemed controlling. Perhaps I appeared demanding. Perhaps I had an unpleasant tone to my voice. Perhaps he simply did not agree with my dishwashing standards. Whatever was the source of his disagreement with me in that moment is not as important to this story as my reaction and subsequent behavior.

I became very upset. First I was upset that he would not do the dishes as I wanted. But then the deeper, insecure issues started to come up as well: *Here I have caused an argument, a fight even. Now he is mad at me. Now he is displeased with me. Now he can and will tell me all the things wrong with me.*

I left the house and walked down our long driveway. This was a common way for me to manage my first bursts of bad feelings. Halfway down the driveway I paced back and forth, sat for a few moments on a bench there, and then headed back to the house. Monty was sitting in the darkened living room watching television. I made a few attempts to clarify my self, explaining and trying to make things somewhat okay again between us.

My efforts did not work. My devoted watching behaviors came into play fairly quickly. In my watching I could see that he was not looking at me. He was watching the television. He would answer my questions with only brief responses. He would not elaborate or converse. My abandonment fears started coming into play. He was, in fact, already leaving me in these moments as he disconnected from our interaction, and my fears of his permanent removal of him self from me enlarged. The existence of the object of my devotion was threatened, and I was losing my self in my fears.

So I took my self on another walk, this time even farther down the driveway and onto the country road. It was dark. I knew I was not going to go far, but I had upset energy that needed to be used. Walking is a good idea in such a case.

A small distance down the road was an old garage that our car mechanic, Keith, used. He repaired our cars well and was fun to talk with about our car problems. We liked Keith a lot. As I got closer to his driveway, I could see through the dark that he had it blocked off with a chain, and on that chain was a sign that said "Closed." I had never seen this before. This was not how Keith closed up his business on a daily basis. I knew this meant something else—perhaps that he was closed for good.

This piece of different, local news allowed me to shift my mood and focus away from being upset with my husband and onto absorbing and announcing this information. I turned and hurried back to the house to tell him what I had learned. I walked back into the house, sat down again in my chair in the darkened room lit only by the television that Monty continued to watch, and proceeded to tell him what I had just found out. He listened to me and engaged in the conversation more than he had before. I watched him as he did so, and I could tell he was again connecting with me enough in that moment to slightly quiet my abandonment fears.

I offered to pop corn, which I knew we enjoyed together. He said sure. I felt better.

To me, this story is about devotion in these ways: I am loyal to my husband, and I allow my loyalty and devotion to become confused with unhealthy attachments and fears of abandonment. As I sink into a blind devotion, it can involve "compelling motives and often attachment to an objective."* Let's look again more carefully at these key words that resound through this story.

Compel means "to drive or urge forcefully or irresistibly; to cause to do or occur by overwhelming pressure."* As I walked up and down our driveway, what I was really doing was trying to find a way to force Monty and me to be okay with each other again after this disagreement. I wanted to fix the situation. I wanted to control how he was being with me. I no longer cared about the dishes. The objective I had become attached to was to not have him leave me. That is the irrational fear out of which my totally devoted self was acting.

Compelled is a good word to hold onto as we learn to differentiate between healthy devotion and insanity. In my state of total devotion, I am compelled to hold onto you, to not let you go, to watch you for reassurance about me and us; most of all, I can be compelled to abandon me so you will not abandon me. If I am not taking care of my self in such moments, I will let go of whatever I want, need, think, or care about just so you will come back to me.

Never mind the dishes that I wanted to have washed. I'll gladly change the subject and fix popcorn if that reestablishes the fine balance I need to feel secure and reassured that the object of my devotion is not

*By permission. From *Merriam-Webster's Collegiate® Dictionary*, 11th Edition ©2012 by Merriam-Webster, Incorporated (www.Merriam-Webster.com).

going away. I'll watch you carefully and obsessively until I am satisfied that you are okay with me, forgetting to consider if *I* am okay with me.

Even as Daisy watches me in the morning, I am fantasizing that she is afraid I am going to leave her and not come back. I have heard that dogs cannot conceptualize that we will return, so when we do come back to them they are delightfully surprised all over again to be in our presence.

Maybe all of my thoughts about Daisy and my leaving are my own projections. To a large extent I am sure they are. When I reassure Daisy I will come home and see her again, I am speaking from my own issues and hopes that the person I am watching with such dedication will not leave me and never come back.

To be so watchful, devoted, and dependent is a shaky way to live.

Lessons Learned

I have learned that devotion can go too far. Watching behaviors are a specific way to notice devotion going too far. Watching itself is tricky, because it involves an external orientation. The act of watching involves me paying attention to things and people outside of my self. I am observing the other person's behaviors, facial expressions, tones, glances, gestures, postures. To a certain extent this is functional and appropriate in terms of cultivating conversations and relationships. But if my codependence allows me to let this external orientation dominate, then I am likely to lose my self.

Remember, I spoke of the value of seeing relationships in terms of a scale or a balance between internal and external orientations. Watching makes us prone to the external. And if we glean potentially negative data from our watching, then we are at even more risk for engaging in an external orientation as we maneuver to attempt to reestablish what we fear we may be losing from the other person.

So I have learned:

Devotion can be a good thing. Loyalty and commitment help us to grow as individuals and in relationships. By being involved in these ways, we can learn more about our self and make changes that enrich and strengthen us. Devotion can help us to have a home base, a set of beliefs and values by which we live. Daisy and I both benefit from being devoted creatures.

I can lose my self in my devotion. In being loyal and committed, it is important for me to consider my self as well. This does not mean that I must always have my way or attend to my needs without consideration of others. It does mean that as I deeply attend to someone else, or, for that matter, some cause or activity, I also connect with me. Is what I am about to choose good for me? Will I feel okay about me and my choices if I am acting out of my devotion? Am I starting to feel compelled to say or do things that may be driven by my devotion? Has my devotion blurred into obsessive watching and checking to protect my self from abandonment by this object of my devotion?

Watch out for my watching. I need to be mindful of my watching behaviors. I need to notice when I am slipping into them and not let my self go too far. This means I stop my self from trying to read others and from trying to guess what they want from me. I need to listen well and respond in ways that are true for me.

I do not really know how others are feeling or what they are thinking unless they tell me. Because of my tendency toward focusing on the other person, I must believe I have exceptional abilities to think and speak for that person and to know what he or she feels and wants. I am wrong. This is not so. I do best by working on knowing *my* internal self and leaving the same to the other person to do for his or her self.

Other people are responsible for themselves. Without sounding too hard-hearted, this means that not only do I not have to guess what they want, but also I do not have to give them what I think they want. My efforts to please and accommodate others can leave me not pleasing or accommodating my self.

It is important for me to be able to express my self to others. If I am losing my self in watching, then I am shifting into a defensive posture, a posture where the goal becomes to not lose the other person. Ironically, in so doing I am losing my self. I must retain my self by consciously remembering my presence, my thoughts, and my feelings, which I want to be able to express.

I can be my self and not be abandoned. As I have braved the waters of codependence recovery, I have challenged my self to test this out, and no one has abandoned me.

This abandonment issue is a bit more complicated than just that last statement. I have also learned that

If someone abandons me because I am true to my self, that person is not someone I want to spend time with.

And, even more importantly,

I do not want to abandon my self. Again, ironically, the greatest abandonment with codependence is that of self-abandonment. When who I am and what I think and do is molded around someone else, then I am in trouble, because I really need that person for my identity, sanity, and security. If I find, cultivate, and treasure my self, I can never be abandoned—as long as I am watchful of my self and am devoted to caring for me in this loving way.

hardworking

"Keep me busy!
Keep me busy!"

Characteristic Described

Defining *hardworking* does not require the dictionary. Most all of us know exactly what that means: works hard. Usually hard workers do thorough and reliable work. They take their work seriously and often do well with both the quantity and quality of their work. They are desirable employees and partners in relationships. They can be depended upon and can be very productive.

I can be this way. To a certain extent these characteristics are very desirable. When our daughter Grace was just four or five years old, she and I were playing in the living room in front of the wood stove, with me on my hands and knees and Grace riding on my back like I was a pony. As we were doing this, Grace said about me, "She's a slow little pony, but she gets the job done." Well, that can just about sum me up. Grace and I have quoted her on this many times over the years. The "slow" part can be true, and I especially like "she gets the job done." I was glad she knew that.

Several years later Grace said, "You can always count on Momma." I treasure that message from Grace. I am glad she could always count on me, and I will do my best to always make that true. At the same time, as I write this statement, I know that there may well be limits on me at times to "always" come through for her. We will be looking at such limits as this chapter proceeds, for hard work *can* go too far, with a price to the individual and to others. A work supervisor of mine many years ago described me as "obsessively overresponsible." I don't think that was a compliment. I think I have been trying for many years to moderate my work style into health. I still am.

As I quote about the border collie in the Preamble, "First and foremost, the border collie is a working dog . . . . Without meaningful work, border collies will become bored and depressed and may develop behavior problems."

"The border collie is a working dog who thrives on having a job to do and a purpose in life."

I love each of those sentences about the border collie. They make me smile every time I read them, because they are so true of the dog, and they can be so true of the codependent. Without meaningful work, I could become depressed and develop behavior problems. I could become irritable and lost, especially if my work has been a primary way in which I define my self. If my job or life purpose is too external to my very self, then without it I risk feeling like nothing. This is broadly expressed here, but that's okay for these budding lessons about "Hardworking."

To clarify, in this chapter I am talking about the general style of hardworking. There are many types of work and jobs that both the border collie and the codependent do. Some of those jobs will be specifically examined in other chapters. Here I am studying the basic quality of hard work no matter what form that work takes.

So what does hard work involve? It is greatly helped by focus, desire, motivation, and interest, and by strength, stamina, and endurance. Hard work can also be facilitated by pride in one's accomplishments and desires to contribute, to fix, and to please.

The border collie is built for this type of hard work. Athleticism is one of its characteristics. Mary Burch describes the border collie as "a well balanced, medium-sized dog of athletic appearance, displaying grace and agility in equal measure with substance and stamina. His hard muscular body has a smooth outline which conveys the impression of effortless movement and endless endurance . . . ."[20] The border collie is bred to perform strenuous work for long periods of time and can cover maximum distance in an efficient manner without tiring.

As for focusing, "Most border collies are intense dogs who can become absolutely focused on a task . . . . There is undoubtedly time for friendship and closeness when the day's work is done, but overall border collies were bred to be focused on work."[21]

Within these descriptions are words that capture the essence of hard work and that I believe, through my experiences, can be true of individuals with codependent styles. Those meaningful words include substance and stamina, effortless movement, endless endurance, energy, eagerness, and absolute focus. As I wrote this list I paused at the inclusion of effortless movement, wondering if it is as true as the other descriptors of hard work, and then I remembered another tale about me from my work.

I was running an adolescent day treatment program in my community. I was the sole employee of the program. I did everything from driving the van for the program to conducting the group therapy there. I remarked to a colleague about my disappointment that I had received no additional funding for the program. She replied to me, "Well, Nancy, you make it look so easy."

"You make it look so easy." I had no idea. I wasn't trying to convey that impression. I was simply doing my job and more, without my awareness or expressed feelings or needs for more help. I was handling whatever came my way, with no expectations for help and no limits on what I would do. I imagine this makes for a good employee and a happy employer, but I am coming to see that it does not necessarily make for a healthy individual.

These tendencies for hard work by the codependent can be understood by looking at several of the core defining features of codependency. In general, our work habits can be seriously influenced by *external focusing,* by our being so intent on the behaviors, opinions, and expectations of others and by obtaining approval and esteem from others that we lose our self. Yes, the work environment can be complex, with many external demands on us. Working for other people, especially, by its nature, involves these external expectations and evaluations of performance accordingly. So if we are inclined toward wanting to accommodate others and usually operate out of an external orientation, then those of us with codependent characteristics will be additionally challenged when it comes to managing our hard work.

This takes us directly to *self-sacrificing,* another defining feature of codependency. Self-sacrificing speaks of putting the needs of others above our own. Sometimes in life this is necessary, but as a general way of operating this can cause us trouble. In terms of our working behaviors specifically, if we consistently overextend our self by ignoring our own needs, believe that we need to take more than our fair share of the responsibilities, and think it is selfish to take care of our self along the way, then our work, our relationships, and our self will suffer.

Many of us by now have heard the caution against self-sacrificing from airline staff. They tell us that in the event of an emergency where the oxygen masks drop down to our faces, we should put on our own oxygen mask first before trying to help the people around us needing our assistance. Put on your own mask first. This is not selfish. This is imperative in order to be able to do the extraordinary work at hand.

And then there is the dynamic of *interpersonal control*. Remembering that this means that we deeply believe that we can fix and control others, let's apply this to hardworking. With such a belief system, this is almost a setup for extra work, extra effort, and extra frustration. Certainly offering to help others can be just fine. The problem comes when we are preoccupied with trying to fix others; when we believe that things will fall apart if we do not tightly manage people and situations; when we think we have to do something so that it will be done correctly; or when we are driven by our deeper need to have everything be under control. With such a list of possible characteristics centered around the issues of control, it is clear how our work behaviors can easily escalate and likely cause us problems if we are operating out of a belief that nothing being asked of us is too much, too far, or too expensive if it achieves the outcome we have designated and desire.

Tales Told

I do not have one specific story to tell you about Daisy and work. She has not grown up on a sheep farm. In fact, she has not grown up on a farm at all. She lives in our small, clapboard house on a creek that runs into a river we can see from our front windows. She has lived these sixteen years in the company of my husband, daughter, and me along with our other dog Eddie, cats, and shorter-lived pets including fish, a canary, mice, and rats. She has had no responsibility for herding or managing any of us.

Early on Grace said that Daisy "ran away from a circus to join a home." She said this in response to the strength and athleticism that Daisy has shown us from the beginning. Clearly she has the genes for beautiful, fast running, for alertness and responsiveness, and for the high energy of the border collie. In her younger years Daisy would stand in place and jump high enough to see out the window in the upper half of a door. In fact, she would do such jumping, in general, to look in her food bowl when someone had it in hand or to see into a car window. She stands up on her hind legs with good balance and has such an endearing prance to her step that it usually prompts me to say, "Daisy, you make me smile."

Daisy's agility has always been clear and impressive. A path runs from our front yard down to the creek and then the river. It winds its way down with a couple of distinct, sharp turns—switchbacks, you could say. When Daisy knows we are going to the river, she will run ahead of us down the path—race down the path, actually—turn sharply at the bottom of the path, and race back up the path to the top and back down again, rushing past us each time and continuing this agile performance of back-and-forth with sharp turns until we are all down at the river. A regret of mine is that I never took Daisy to formal agility training. Her potential is so clear, her abilities so strong, her energy so good. She is a working dog waiting for a job. She may have run away from a circus to join a home, but she's still built for work.

So what work has Daisy taken on, living this simple river cottage life? Three jobs I can readily observe through her behaviors are providing companionship, greeting, and protecting. These three jobs are all related in that they center around relationships as her work, especially Daisy's relationship with us, her family, and, even more specifically, Daisy's relationship with me. As I said earlier, my husband and daughter both agree that without any doubt I am Daisy's main relationship. So I am the one who is the most pronounced beneficiary of her work as a companion, greeter, and protector—though I believe she acts protectively for all of us.

As a companion for me, Daisy is excellent. She takes this work seriously and with dedication. She is often in the same room as me. When I move from place to place in the house, she notices and follows me. When I say let's go on a walk or down to the river, she's ready to go—not just to go, but to be with me there. I am glad for her good company and deeply appreciate her loving work as one of my favorite companions.

As a greeter, Daisy is outstanding. Here's how it usually happens: When I arrive back at our home, as soon as I am parking my car in our driveway, Monty and the dogs come out of the house to greet me. Often I can hear Monty say, "Daisy, Nancy's home!" If I am not yet completely out of the car, Daisy will jump up to see me through the car window, or as I open the door, she will come up to me even as I still sit in my seat. And then she takes off with her amazing spontaneous display of agility and enthusiasm, running around the car, running around our hilly yard, running around buckets of rainwater we collect. She has great speed and makes sharp turns. We cheer her on and she performs with even more pride and enthusiasm, strength and agility. In this greeting job of hers she offers a full extension of her self, which continues as we all come into the house with Daisy doing a modified running from room to room and leaping from rug to rug. I then give Daisy a treat and, feeling quite welcomed in my own home, I say, "You are such a good working dog."

In these two jobs, companionship and greeting, I have no great tales of Daisy's work going too far. I am sure she could carry them to extremes. For example, her work as a companion could have her unable to be separate from me without becoming a maniac. Or her greeting behaviors could spiral out of control, with her running madly out into the darkness and getting lost or injuring her self. These extremes have not happened in these jobs, but in terms of her work as a protector, Daisy can go too far.

Let's call this tale "The Man with the Hat."

Daisy barks unnecessarily at strangers, and for the most part anyone outside of our immediate household is a stranger to Daisy. So whether they are friends pulling up in our yard to visit or canoeists briefly stopped on our delta, Daisy barks at them. And she doesn't just bark. She runs toward them barking. She never goes all the way up to them, nor does she nip or bite. But her posturing is aggressive and protective of her territory. We have never been able to successfully train Daisy to not do this.

Daisy particularly has trouble with men wearing hats—all men and any type of hat. Early in Daisy's life with us this became clear. Family friends came to visit us: a mother, a father, and two young children. Grace was very young, too. They had come especially so the children could play together. The father had on a baseball cap, which he always wears. Daisy did not like this one bit. She barked at him forcefully as he got out of the car. We disciplined her, she reluctantly quieted, and we all went into our house.

We gathered in the living room to visit, and Daisy again noticed this man with a hat in her space and launched into her barking posture. We tried a number of things to quiet her, including firm commands, having our guest briefly remove his cap to let her see him better, and removing Daisy from the room.

None of our efforts were fully successful in helping Daisy to know that she did not have to protect us from this man, our friend, our welcomed guest. Daisy had it in her head that this was a job she needed to do, and she poured herself into it without any regard for reason, for limits, for listening to us, or for the reality of the situation. Truly, she was ridiculous. At times she would get quiet and rest, but then, as soon as she was again aware of this man with the hat still in our living room, she was on the job—a job she had taken on her self and was determined to do no matter what.

*   *   *   *   *

I, too, take on jobs that I determine must be done no matter what.

As I was thinking about a tale about me and hard work, I considered writing about my being the "Last One Home in Rockbridge County." I work in my office four days each week, and those are very long days. Granted, some of the hours of those days are spent exercising and taking dance classes and occasionally having lunch with friends, but most of those hours are spent working. When I drive home at 9:30 or 10:00 at night, there is almost no one else on the road during my twenty-five-minute trip. Many houses are dark, with people obviously having called it quits and gone to bed. Likely they had supper, cleaned up, and relaxed with television or a book before turning off the lights, while I am just going home. More and more I realize something is wrong with my picture, this picture of me, my work, and my day. I tell my self that I balance this work schedule out by having a three-day weekend each week. That helps, for sure, but I believe I am fooling my self and that my hard work, which has me closing up Rockbridge County Mondays through Thursdays, is looking suspiciously like it is going too far and merits my self-awareness and self-intervention.

I had thought I would say more about this questionable work pattern of mine, and then I remembered a tale from my high school days that fully illustrates these dynamics of hard work that can go too far—hard work that involves enthusiasm, energy, intensity, purpose, drive . . . and collision. Let's call this tale "High School Drama."

I was a real go-getter in school. I got excellent grades and was involved in many school activities. Seems I was building my resume even then, though not with direct awareness. In the ninth grade I started high school, and for some reason I was in charge of the freshman class float for our homecoming parade. I believe I had this job because I was vice president of our freshman class. I was also a junior varsity cheerleader, which was a dream come true for me.

Even today I don't know much about creating a float for a parade from beginning to end, so it's hard to imagine how I had any idea of what I was doing then. Nevertheless, I did it—practically single-handedly.

The homecoming event was at the City Stadium in Richmond, Virginia. It was the fall of 1966. We constructed the floats at the stadium during the day, where they paraded around the football field prior to the game that night. The plan for this day of the parade was that we would make the float, then I would go home, change into my cheerleading outfit, and return to the stadium to ride on a convertible in the parade with the other junior varsity cheerleaders—a tall order for this hardworking fourteen-year-old.

The construction of the float was difficult. Out of our freshman class of 500, three people, including me, showed up to work on it. I remember being frustrated and disappointed, but needing to be the one to take it all on if it was to happen. So that is what I did. I don't remember the theme or details of the float; I do remember feeling like it didn't look like much and not being very proud of it except that it had gotten done. In order for it to be finished, our little band of three had to work way too close to the start time of the evening events.

I rushed home to change clothes and get ready to be in the parade, my premiere as a junior varsity cheerleader. My dear high school boyfriend drove me home and back, with each way taking at least thirty minutes of city driving. I was rushing. I felt pressed. I felt tense. I felt mad. I had worked so hard, so long, and was becoming resentful of everyone else in the world who wasn't. As we were driving back down The Boulevard to the stadium, I remember thinking, "No one better give me a hard time about arriving just in time to get on the cheerleaders' car." I was all wound up and uncharacteristically looking for a fight. I was tired, late, and mad, mad, mad.

I got there just in time to get on the hood of the convertible for our happy parading. And sure enough, one of my least favorite members of our squad said to me in her condescending voice, "Nancy, where have you been? We've been all ready and you're holding us up!" Though in that moment I knew that was almost true, what I knew even better was that I had been working my butt off that day for this homecoming show and she had not! I had been running around trying to get a ridiculous amount of work done and she had not! Instead, she likely had been home getting all dolled up to look pretty on our convertible ride, while I felt like I hardly had my uniform on straight. I was sick of her and the whole day, and I told her so in no uncertain terms, there in the lights of the stadium, with the band playing and our entire squad present.

Time required that I shut up and get on the car and join in the enthusiastic cheers as we traveled the track around the football field. "Go! Panthers! Go!" I was smiling, energetic, clapping, looking like I was having such fun, being such a positive model of school spirit and citizenship. I knew this was all appearance for me at this time. I knew I had just had a collision and was reeling from that inside my self.

As soon as the parade was over, our cheerleading sponsor was waiting for me and took me directly to the large public bathroom under the stadium. She, too, had been at the car when I fell apart, and with great sternness, she asked to know what in the world was wrong with me. By now I had turned into a heap of tears and remorse for my behavior. My anger had been expressed. I told her about my frustrating day of work, of the pressures I had felt, and of all the running around I had done. I know now that I was also telling her that I was so busy doing so much for so many other people that I did not have time for my self, nor did any of these other people I had done so much for show any appreciation, understanding, or even awareness.

Sound familiar? It does to me. It sounds like codependence experienced and expressed by my fourteen-year-old self. Not only was I overextending my self in work, but those behaviors were tangled with expectations of others as well as self-neglect.

My conversation with our cheerleading sponsor ended okay. She listened well, acknowledged this was uncharacteristic behavior on my part, and let me go back and join the squad with no consequences other than a clear admonition to never let this happen again.

Forty-six years later I am telling you this tale as a way to continue to work on not letting this happen again.

Lessons Learned

And so I am learning:

Work is good. Work is important. Work gets necessary things done, fun things accomplished, and creative efforts launched. Work can feed me, both literally and figuratively, and enrich my life. I enjoy work. I enjoy activity and productivity. I enjoy being full of ideas of things I want to do for my self and others. And I enjoy doing those things. I can fill every corner of my day with these various forms of work that I enjoy. I have the endurance and stamina to keep going. And often I do. This is not necessarily bad, but I am also learning:

Work can go too far. My drive, purpose, and productivity can turn into obsession if I am not mindful and honest with my self. Just like Daisy and her incessant barking at the man with the hat, I can set my own work agenda and fall headlong into its execution and completion, come hell or high water. I can ignore important cues within my self and outside of my self that say to stop or take a break. In so doing I can damage my self, my important relationships, and, ironically, the task at hand. When we are packing for a family trip and are running around extremely busy with many jobs to do, we have learned that if we are not careful, this hard work to get out the door can result in tension and arguments and make us not even want to get in the car and go on a vacation with each other when this preparation work is done.

Be careful of attaching expectations of others to my work. If I am working predominantly for the approval of others, I may well be setting my self up for disappointment or anger. My work may not evoke the responses I want, and then I may feel that this lack of external response negates the work I have done.

I want to do my work for my own pleasure and approval, even if it has been assigned to me by others. When my boss or family member has asked something of me, I do have to consider the specific needs of the assignment they have given me, *and* I also want to anchor my self in my work, quieting all of the external questions and worries so that I can think and be with me and the work itself. This is the way I can do my best work and feel good about it.

Be careful of my own demanding self. Sometimes our drive for approval of our work is not only about seeking that approval from others, but about demanding it of our self. Our perfectionism and need to control can make work extra-arduous and time-consuming. I know this directly. Not only do I like to get things done, but I like them done my way. Whether I like to admit that or not, it is true, and my owning it is essential to my changing it, to my being able to find a better balance for my self with work.

I do this to my self. I am the one making my list of work that is too long to be completed that day. I am the one who presses on to the next item, simultaneously rushing and demanding that the things on my list be done just right. I am the one ignoring hunger, fatigue, and time. I am the one barking despite internal and external messages to stop.

I don't have to do it all right now. Even if I have a long list of things I want to do in a day or in a week, I need to teach my self that I don't have to do them all right now. I know I have some obsessive-compulsive aspects to my self that press me to get closure on as many things as I can, as soon as I can. I know that behind that obsessive-compulsive drive is my anxiety, which believes it will be quieted in an effective way by having all of these things done. I know this is not so. I know this drive in me to get all of this done is an unhealthy part of my self that can be a bottomless pit. There will always be more I want to do, more to add to my list. So it is imperative that I work with my self to have a realistic grasp of what I can do and keep learning to manage that part of me that keeps adding to my list.

Some things I don't even have to do at all. Imagine that: some things don't have to be done at all. As a hardworking codependent, this is an exciting and challenging lesson to absorb. You mean I don't have to find just the right napkins for our dinner party tonight? You mean white napkins will work just fine? You mean I don't have to make an extra trip to town to buy more orange juice? You mean we can live another couple of days without it? Small details like these can really add to my workload, and I am understanding the need to let some things go, to not have to have everything just like I want it to be, because that is not possible and/or my overworking to make these things happen will drive me and others crazy.

My to-do list is not a life sentence. I still believe in lists. They help me to get things out of my head, and they provide a road map for me as I prioritize the items on the list and define subtasks needed to get the jobs done. But we have to be cautious about the power of "The List." People tell me they love to check items off their list. This is okay unless we become so driven to check off items that we lose track of our very self. And then there was the person who described her self as living her life off a list. At least she was aware of this behavior and the way it was dominating and controlling her and limiting her fuller participation in her life. So as I make my to-do list, I want to remember that it is only a list, a guide, a reminder—not an absolute sentence handed down to me that must be done fully, immediately, and perfectly before anything else is possible.

I can ask for help. Yes, my hero role has me believing that I must be the one to do things, that there is no one else who can do the job, that asking for help is weak. And yes, my perfectionism and need to control can make it challenging to give jobs to others, because the job won't be done just as I want it to be done. My awareness of these characteristics of my self is important, then, to my intervening on my own behalf and changing these old patterns in the present moment. Who could help? What could they help with? Who might even want to help? Who has offered to help? What resources have been offered to me that I am not accepting and that could lighten my load and my spirit?

Everyone doesn't work like me. Now I am not asking for an award for the way and amount I work. Though Daisy and I are both intense workers by nature, no one should reward us for working to the point of self-destruction. The way I work is, in general, good and useful, but I can overdo it. And as I overdo it, I am inclined to become judgmental of people who are not working the way I do: How dare he take a break! How can she put that off until tomorrow? What does he mean, "That's good enough"? Just because these are not words and phrases immediately in my vocabulary does not mean that these are not good ways to work. In fact, these are probably strong concepts to add to my repertoire in order to find a better balance for my self with work.

I can ruin my body. Daisy and I do have strength, stamina, and endurance. We can work long hours, employing our tireless and high-energy bodies. And I do know I can overdo this. It's hard to think very well if I am hungry or tired. When I am tired I become irritable and unhappy. I become impatient and critical. Long-term wear and tear like this can cause diagnosable psychological and medical conditions. Stress is a word used by many these days to describe this condition of taking on too much and then feeling the consequences of doing so through problems with mood, sleep, weight loss or gain, digestion, or immune deficiencies, to name a few. It is imperative that I be mindful of my basic biological needs and respond to them in a serious and meaningful way as I make my way through my day's work.

I can ruin my relationships. If I am working too hard for too long, I start not being my best self. Not only do I become worn out, but I can also, as I said above, become irritable, critical, and demanding of others. They are not doing enough! They are not appreciating me enough! They are not as good as I am! They are lazy and worthless! Such messages, whether I say them to my self or out loud, are very damaging to our relationships with others. Daisy's barking relentlessly at the man with the hat certainly did not help her to win him over. My barking at others won't help my relationships, either. In fact, such carrying on by me as a result of my overworking can only cause distance and mistrust in these relationships affected by my work style. In order for me to have healthy, meaningful relationships with others, I need to be able to set my work aside, respond to my basic needs, and then approach those I love with a sociability that is warm, friendly, and not full of the task-oriented, production-driven style with which I can lead.

I can ruin my day. I really want to remember this. I hate it when I work so hard, finish what I wanted to do, and then am so tired or frazzled that I cannot enjoy it. This can occur with doing yard work or giving a party. In other words, I can have this pattern whether the work is a mundane job or a fun activity. I don't want to do this to my self. I don't want to do this to others who may be affected by my exhaustion. I want to balance the assignments I give to my self so that

I can enjoy them as I do them, enjoy them when they are done, and enjoy the people in my life who are around me as all of this is going on. When the day's work is over, I want to be glad for my work, my relationships, and my life.

I can ruin my spirit. Built into all of this talk about overworking is my neglect of spirit. When I make my lists and take off with my must-do jobs, I am likely operating without any connection to my higher power. I am in my ripping-and-tearing mode and probably trying to control things I cannot control. I may not even notice this neglect of spirit. I am too busy deciding what needs to be done and how to do it. It is thus very important for me to remember what I am learning:

My spirituality is an essential resource for helping me to manage my hard work. Connecting with my breath helps me to connect with my spirituality. My mindfulness and twelve-step practice have helped this to be an almost automatic path for me. As I reconnect with my breath, this is an opening that then connects me with my higher power and all the wonderfulness that comes from letting go of so much of my drive. I can think better. I can feel some spaciousness between my self and my tasks. I can make healthier decisions about what to do and what not to make my self do now. We have all heard that when we are pressed we should stop and take deep breaths. Well, there's tons of truth to that, not only because of the healthy pause it creates for us but also because of the possibilities it creates within us for the entrance of spirit. I'm just not sure how to teach this to Daisy.

serving

*"Is there anything
I can do for you?"*

Characteristic Described

Codependents are known to be helpers, and this chapter is about our helping behaviors, our desire to fix, take care of, and give to others. It happens that I have chosen to use the word *serve* to talk about this important category of characteristics. Serving is a way the border collie can be described, and I believe it is a lovely way to consider our helping behaviors and their ability to range from useful and important to damaging.

In the previous chapter, I wrote about hard work as a general style for the border collie and the codependent. Serving is a particular form of hard work. It is one of the jobs we choose to do. It is the type of item we put on our to-do lists: help, give, take care of. As with the border collie, it is our nature to want to do this type of work, and we do it well.

In its basic, healthy form, serving means that we are providing something that is needed or desired, we are answering the needs of others, and/or we are offering services that benefit or help. In order to serve, we have to be aware of the needs of others and give of our self in order to meet those needs. Often healthy serving involves our giving freely with no expectations of something coming back to us for our efforts.

As you have probably come to expect I will say, serving can go too far. As I was preparing to write this chapter, I realized that closely related to the word *serve* is the word *servant*. Servants wait on other people and are expected to give both service and respect to their superiors. The superior is likely to have hired the servant, to have power and control over him or her, and to treat him or her as the superior wishes. The servant, sadly enough, is left to accept the treatment and continue giving despite the external circumstances of the work. Because of this treatment, servants may have limited awareness of their own self and serious limitations on their ability to express and act on behalf of their self.

My experience is that if I am not careful, my serving can shift from healthy to the edges of losing my self in the giving that I am doing. This is where codependence comes into the story. Codependents are often very responsible individuals, and they get a sense of purpose through relationships. Both of these characteristics can lead us from serving to servitude, a lack of freedom to pursue one's own life.

My being responsible for whatever I am responsible for—at home, at work, in relationships, in organizations—is just fine. Taking on responsibilities is an important part of growing up and maturing. Taking on responsibilities within the limits of my personal resources and values is admirable and necessary to a successful life. Taking on more than my fair share of responsibilities becomes unfair to my self and to others. Placing others ahead of my self on a regular basis as I serve will inevitably become a problem. Believing that I must give of my self until I am successful in making things better for others can have no end for me and sell me into the servitude of which I speak.

Having a sense of purpose through relationships is also a valuable asset in life. Enjoying the company of others, learning from them, and creating memories together certainly adds to the meaning of living. The problem comes when our entire sense of self becomes dependent on being needed in these relationships. If our sense of satisfaction or adequacy is based primarily on the extent to which we are able to serve others, this can be a fragile place to live. If our sense of worth comes primarily from being needed for our guidance and help offered to others, then again we are on shaky ground with our self, as this is being dependent on things outside of our self for our mental health.

These codependent characteristics that can lead us from serving to servitude are three of the defining features of codependence. Once again we are seeing the effects of *external focusing,* this focusing on others with an ultimate intent to obtain approval and esteem. If my sense of self is deeply rooted in wanting to help others and I am unable to succeed at doing so, then I may feel depressed and useless and lost. *Self-sacrificing* can play a large part here as well, with the neglect of my own needs in order to meet the needs of others. If I do put the needs of others, including family and friends, ahead of my own needs on a regular basis, then my health and happiness will decline in proportion to my self-neglect and ultimately disable my ability to serve others. Woven into all of this serving that can go too far is *interpersonal control,* my belief that I can fix and control others if I persist in my giving, fixing, and caretaking.

There are those words that are the title of the continuum I spoke of previously: giving, fixing, and caretaking. Really, all of these words are forms of serving, and I refer you back to that section for a detailed reminder of specific behaviors that are included in our serving efforts, remembering that at one end of the continuum offering and suggesting are okay, and at the other end they cause problems for all parties involved. The codependent may become a servant to the other person and/or the other person may come to feel indentured to the codependent. Either way or both ways, this is not a healthy way for either party to live freely.

In fact, this is the heart of codependence as I more deeply understand it: If I serve you, I feel good, and if in my doing this you become dependent on me, I feel even better. Then, in reality, we are both indentured; I am your servant, you are dependent on me, and no one escapes to their own life.

Tales Told

Mary Burch and Daisy both have helped me to see the many ways the border collie serves: herding, protecting, and providing companionship, to name a few. The border collie is very attentive to the moods, desires, and expectations of its owner and is ready to respond to what it understands that person wants. It wants to serve. It is ready to serve. It is its nature to serve.

Further into her book on border collies, Mary Burch says that she has found that there are some lesser-known characteristics of this breed, one of which is honesty. She elaborates on this feature by telling a little story that she entitles "Their Brothers' Keepers"—a story about honesty and serving.

> "Some border collies will watch other dogs engaging in inappropriate activities and report the misbehavior to an owner. One evening around Christmastime, my bedroom door flew open and in rushed my border collie with a wide-eyed, agitated look on his face. He wanted me to come and see what was happening. Downstairs, under the Christmas tree, my Welsh springer spaniel was quietly opening all of the Christmas presents."

Burch explains that this desire of the border collie "to 'tattle' on the other dog probably evolved from the breed's necessity to be able to alert a shepherd with the message, 'Come and look; something's not right here'" [22]

And that is just what Daisy did the day she helped us to find Eddie, our black lab mix. This is a tale of Daisy's serving by offering me the same message: "Come look! Something's not right!"

It was a Saturday afternoon on October 18, 2003. I had been working in our yard, clearing brush on a terrace that runs above and along our creek. Daisy had been outside with me, keeping me company and doing her own wandering around the yard. Fairly near to me, Daisy started barking with intent. She was facing toward the creek, which is also the same direction as the railroad that runs along the river in front of our house. She barked and barked, putting her whole self into this message she was relaying: "Something is not right!"

I squatted down beside her and tried to see whatever it was that she was seeing. I could not see anything. We were looking at a wooded, brushy bank on the other side of our creek bed, and so identifying something in that natural thicket was not easy. Daisy continued to bark, and I continued to try to understand her message with no success—two border collies on alert and ready for action.

I decided to put Daisy in our house so I could look more closely. With the railroad nearby, I did not want Daisy to follow me as I moved in that direction. As I put her in the house, I alerted my husband and daughter to the fact that Daisy was really trying to tell us about something out there, and I was going to check it out further.

I walked out the front door, down our driveway, and to the railroad tracks. There, lying on the tracks, yes, on the tracks, was a black dog leaning against one of the rails. I was not sure what to do, not knowing if the dog was friendly, hurt, or mean. So I walked closer to it and squatted down to speak to it. As I was doing this, Monty and Grace came out to join me. Grace had been getting ready to go to her school's homecoming dance, and so she had on a fancy dress as she made her way out to this event on the tracks. They had left Daisy in the house for this part of the story.

While I only felt safe squatting somewhat near to the dog, Grace made an accurate judgment that she could approach him more closely. Almost within reach of him, Grace invited him to get up and come—which he did! It was immediately noticeable that something was wrong with his back right leg, as he held it up and would not use it at all. He was also very skinny.

Monty, Grace, and I encouraged him to follow us into our yard, and just as he did so, I remember saying, "Hello, Eddie." He had no tags on. I did not know that his name was Eddie, but it came to me as we walked together for the first time that this was who he was. We slowly walked up to our front porch where Eddie lay back down, obviously worn out.

Our party expanded by two. Before Grace had come out to the tracks, she had called her best friend, Amy, who lived three miles up the river from us and who was also getting ready for the dance. Amy drove into the yard just as we got to the porch and got out of her car, looking fine in her homecoming attire. Amy is quite a dog lover and is very good with them, as you will recall from the Regional Fair story. So her presence added to the loveliness of this welcoming of Eddie.

We let Daisy come out of the house. We did this with caution and paying great attention, since we had no idea how it would be as these two dogs came together. But both of them were gracious toward each other and have been ever since.

We called the emergency telephone number for our veterinarian and asked the person on call what we could feed this stray, malnourished dog. We gave him some water and a bit of food, and chose to let him come into our house. I think we knew already that he would be staying. We have never been more than a one-dog family, but things changed for us in those moments.

Grace and Amy went off to the dance. Monty and I and Daisy and Eddie settled in for the night. The evening passed without incident for any of us. We continued to notice that Eddie would not use his back right leg, even when he wanted to try to see what was on our counters for food. Daisy went about her own little life.

In the middle of that same night I got up to go to the bathroom and found Eddie all stretched out and lying on his back on our burgundy loveseat. We do not allow our dogs to get up on the furniture, but I refused to disturb Eddie from his great rest that night. With food in his belly and a home surrounding him, I could only imagine how wonderfully relieved he felt.

Our veterinarian saw Eddie the next Monday. We found out that he did have a broken leg, and she said he had likely not eaten for three weeks. Over the next three months, we cared for Eddie's leg so that he regained full use of it, and we fed him and loved him and made him our own.

And all of this is thanks to Daisy for her service in letting me know something was not right in our yard. I know that through this behavior Daisy was serving me. Interestingly enough, though, in the long run she also served Eddie, who was healed and given a home. We have no idea what would have happened to Eddie, whether he would have been hit by a train, which did come by shortly after we invited him off of the tracks. Daisy really did serve as her brother's keeper. Maybe Daisy did know there was a dog over there when she was barking. Maybe she did know that dog needed help. We won't ever know these types of details.

We do know that Daisy provided an important service that changed all of our lives, including her own. I do not believe that Daisy overfunctioned as she served in this story. She noticed, responded, offered of her self, and then let go, even to the extent that she was able to allow this new dog to live with her. Her service to me allowed our service to Eddie.

And so it is with healthy serving. We offer what we can, when we can, and how we can, and we do not necessarily ever know the full impact of our service as it radiates out into the world. In general, I like to operate with this deep belief that we are all interconnected, and what I offer within my healthy resources can ripple out in ways I will never know. But when my serving gets out of the bounds of what I can competently and freely offer, I can get in trouble with my self, with others, and with this lovely flow of healthy service such as Daisy's. I can become a frustrated, resentful servant, and the joy of serving can be lost.

*　*　*　*　*

I have done this on more than one occasion, this serving in excess of my healthy bounds. I have done it many, many times, in fact, in small and large ways. Two larger ways have come to my mind as I have found my way here to this tale of my self.

Rather than tell you a specific tale, I have decided to tell you about "My Pattern." I can fall into a pattern relative to serving/helping/giving if I am not careful and mindful. As I tell you about this pattern, I am thinking about my involvement as an adult in two particular long-term activities. One of those activities was a full-time, paid job. The other activity involved volunteering in a community service project. I spent five years at the paid job, and my volunteer work spanned more than four years.

My pattern begins with my being very excited about whatever

it is that I have been asked to do. Note already the word *asked* to do. Codependents do love to feel needed, and to be asked to do something is a great start! So whether I have been asked to do something because I have been hired or I have been asked to do something because I have a particular talent with it, I am eager and ready to serve.

I bring much good energy and many good ideas to my work. I research. I plan. I engage others. I work with whatever resources come my way. I am prepared for whatever I have been asked to do: teach, drive, counsel, create, coach, support. I am eager to offer what I know and what I have prepared. I am reliable. I do not take time off. As Grace said about me when she was a child, "You can always count on Momma." Well, that's part of my pattern. And there is really nothing wrong with that . . . up to a point.

Much time can go by with my functioning in the above way—enthusiastic, engaged, and giving. I believe all is well for me as I do this, and then I start having some additional feelings that are different from the ones I have been describing:

- When no one from the organization ever comes to see how things are going at my program, I am hurt and surprised.
- When I learn that the new budget does not include any additional funding for my program, I am mad and stunned.
- When the organization moves my office and program area while I am on vacation, I am mad and hurt and surprised.
- When I am asked to take on more participants in my program with no additional resources, I am mad and surprised.
- When I have prepared for an activity as I was

asked to do and the person in charge takes over my time and space with no warning or acknowledgment of doing so, I feel mad and hurt and minimized.

- When I am forgotten, whether it is being left off a meeting agenda or a program listing or not being included in future planning, I feel hurt and unimportant.

With this list in mind, you can see how my pattern involves moving from feeling good and engaged in my service to feelings of anger and hurt. It is interesting to note how often I wrote "surprised" as a feeling as well. I believe that I felt surprised because I was happily doing my helping and giving and was not paying enough attention to how I was really feeling about how much I was giving and doing, nor was I paying attention to what additional help and support I might need. It wasn't until that help and support were not offered that I felt my need. The paid job was the same one where someone said to me about my work there, "You make it look so easy." Who would know I needed more help? And when I left the community service work, the person in charge said, "I am very surprised you want to quit." They did not know I had reached my limits on my service there.

Another feeling that emerges from the above list is "minimized" or "not important." I trust that as I began this work, I was not doing it for credit, fame, or fortune. I believe I was doing it for the love of my work and what I have to offer. Though I was not seeking appreciation and recognition, there is no doubt that at some level I needed to at least be remembered, and in both of these situations I felt forgotten. Recognizing that this contrast between excellent service and being forgotten is not good for me, I stopped my work in each of these activities. I was able to do so in comfortable, natural ways as my life changed and new opportunities came my way. The important thing was that I was able to realize in both cases that my service was out of balance with my resources as well as the resources each of these organizations could offer me, and so I was ready and able to stop when I needed to stop.

As I look at the two tales that back up "My Pattern," I realize that things were not horrible in either case. Things could have gotten a lot worse, with more demands on my time and energy and less coming back to me. I could have been assigned jobs I did not want or hours I did not want, or been publicly humiliated in more direct ways. Nevertheless, my service was traveling down the continuum from healthy to not good for me. I was not yet a full servant, but I was feeling taken for granted and knew that more and more was being asked of me with less coming back my way for the sustenance necessary to thrive. Yes, we codependents can work for very little praise and appreciation, but at some point I know I don't like to feel invisible.

Lessons Learned

With these tales in mind, I have learned:

Serving is good, useful, and important. There is no doubt that being helpful and offering our self to others is valuable. It is a natural thing to do. When we see someone with a difficult situation or expressing a problem, it makes sense that we want to help. Serving others helps them and can serve us as well, giving us positive feelings of connection and usefulness. We can all benefit by healthy service.

Notice my self as I serve. We can become so focused on what we are offering to others—what to offer, how to offer, when to do what—that we forget to check in with our self and what may be best for us as we give to others. I am sure this is one reason I put Daisy in the house while I went to look further for what was causing her to bark so intensely. I am sure I was afraid that if I let her walk with me toward the railroad tracks where we found Eddie, she would be paying no attention to her self and get harmed in some way while she was on this mission of service.

Speak up for my self. As I notice my self, there will probably be things that I need to express to others. When I look back at my pattern, I see my self not being aware of how I was moving down my continuum from healthy service to feelings of disappointment and anger. Without that awareness, I definitely could not have spoken up for my self. As I notice how I am feeling and what I am thinking as I am giving/fixing/caretaking, then I can say things like "No, I can't take on any more," or "We won't be able to do that unless I have more money," or "If I put my time into creating that, I'd like to know that my work will really be used." I know this speaking up for our self can be a challenge for those of us with fears of displeasing others and/or even losing our job. However, if we are thoughtful, clear, and what I call neutral in our tone, then this speaking up can be done in a way that honors both our self and the person to whom we are speaking. To help you further, these topics of pleasing and fear will be addressed more completely in upcoming chapters.

Ask for help when needed. Certainly this is an extension of speaking up for our self. It is its own category of speaking up. As we notice how we are doing with our serving, we may feel like "I just can't do this all my self" or "Someone needs to come in here and help." Though the tales I worked from in this chapter are work-related, all of these dynamics can apply as well to life in our home and our service there. So if I am feeling like I need some help, it is likely that I really do, and all involved will benefit by my requesting that help in the same ways that I suggested we speak up in general—thoughtful, clear, neutral. Often codependents do not like to ask for help. In fact, this trait can run deep as we take on more than is good for us. I noticed this trait in Daisy recently as well. Monty and I were camping in the Adirondacks by Lake Eaton. We were on a walk around the edge of the lake with Daisy and Eddie. We were at one particular place where a very large tree was blocking our way. The dogs could not climb over it without our help. We lifted Eddie over without incident. When we reached down to pick up Daisy, she grumbled loudly and gently fought to get out of the hold Monty had on her simply to lift her, then a fifteen-year-old dog, over a gigantic tree. As we walked on, I said to Monty about Daisy's resistance, "I think she feels undignified having to ask for help." Do I feel undignified having to ask for help?

Say yes to help offered. And then there are those situations where someone has said, "How can I help you?" or "Why don't I do such-and-such so you can go do such-and-such?" I have learned to pay attention when this type of offer is being made and not ignore or reject it. In fact, I have learned to see this as a spiritual blessing in that moment, a gift for sure, and I want to be able to stop my self and consider real, useful ways I can respond with a "yes" to the offer.

Be aware of whether I am offering my service genuinely and freely. This is not to say that my service always has to be genuinely and freely offered, but it is a reminder to me to be aware of whether I *really* want to help, and whether I have any hopes of something in particular coming from the service I do. When I am helping because I want to and have no ties to the outcome, the pleasure of my service can be great, and I am not as likely to move down the continuum of serving from "OK" to "Going Too Far" because I am not striving to make something happen through my service other than the act itself.

If I have expectations of something coming back to me, I need to know it. If I am hoping that my hard work will get me a promotion, I want to be aware of that. If I am hoping that the board will give me more funding if I accept more people into my program, I need to be aware of that. If I am hoping that being cooperative with someone means they will be cooperative with me and my ideas, I need to be aware of that. These types of expectations can be slightly hidden from our awareness as we proceed with what we do, and yet they can be very powerful as they come to light, too often because we are not getting back what we hoped to get. Bringing such expectations to my awareness enables me to decide if I want to let them go or discuss their possibilities with the other person(s) involved.

Get real: know what I can expect from others. As an extension of the previous lesson, not only do I want to be aware of my expectations of others, I also want to be aware if my expectations have any basis in reality. If I know that our budget is going to be cut, then how realistic is it for me to hope my program will get more money? If I know the person in charge repeatedly changes plans, even plans that we have completed and are ready to go, then how realistic is it for me to expect that what I am ready and waiting to do will necessarily be what we do at all—even if I have been enthusiastic and workable through the process? Getting real can be painful as we let go of reasonable hopes and plans, and it can free us from the potential tangles of unrealistic beliefs of "If I do _____, then they will do _____."

Bad feelings from serving serve no one. If we go back to the original idea of serving, we remember that serving in and of itself can be rewarding and a good way to contribute positively to our life here on this earth. If, however, in our serving we start to feel tangled by our expectations or we are giving in excess of our personal resources, then the serving will begin to not be good for anyone. Serving has become a chore, a requirement, a resentment, and none of us are kindly served by such experiences. In such circumstances it might be better for everyone not to continue with that particular act of service, or at least to take a break and see if the good spirit of giving and helping may be found again by restoring some balance in efforts and expectations.

I do not want to become a servant. As I started this chapter, I wrote of the possible slide from serving to becoming a servant. I know that I do not want to give to the point of being inconsiderately controlled by someone else. I do not want to put my self into a situation where my sense of self is dependent on the way someone else treats me. I know that when people ask me repeatedly to do things they could do but won't do, I become resentful. When I am the one up and doing work while others are doing whatever they please, the servant factor starts to show up for me, and I don't like that feeling. And neither do the people around me, because my poor attitude about this becomes clear to all. Though I like to help, I do not make a good servant.

I do not want someone else to be dependent on my service. The very deep part of codependence feeds on being needed by others, by encouraging the dependence of others. This is often not in our awareness as we give, help, and fix. But it is there, and being mindful of this part of our self is an essential part of our recovery. My twelve-step program advises us not to do things for others that they can do for themselves. That's an important guide to help me not make someone else dependent on me. My recovery has taught me that I want others to grow and become their own strong, individuated selves, and then, for those of us who have strong, individuated selves, the potential for us to have healthy relationships is dramatically increased.

Leave/stop if I need to and can. In a previous lesson, I mentioned that sometimes we may need to stop our giving or take a break from it if our frustration and resentment are growing. I think this is important to remember and to give our self permission to do. It is usually easy to know when these feelings are showing up. We may be mumbling to our self, "Why can't anyone else do that?" "I already took my turn doing that!" or "I don't want to do that!" These are straightforward messages to our self. Our assignment is to listen to them and do something to honor them. I am trying to do this. So when I am saying such exclamations to my self, I try to find a way to let go of the task either for that moment or for good. I like that phrase: *for good.* We use it to mean that that is the end; we will do it no more. But note the embedded message. It says to me that stopping in such a case will be good for everyone involved. Not more, but less, is what is good for us all when serving is going too far.

If I can't stop, then find ways to cut back on my giving so as to create a better balance. Certainly there are situations where we are serving and we can't stop. This could be true with helping family members or at a job that we cannot afford to leave. Sometimes we can't stop our service to a committee or board until we have finished our tasks or term. Even if we can't stop or leave, it is important to notice when we are starting to go too far in our giving and to make adjustments accordingly. This means to consider how I can give less time, not add on more tasks, not volunteer to do one more thing, even if it is the best idea on earth. Simultaneously, this finding a better balance may include doing something separate from this demanding service to restore my energy and spirit. What might that be? What feeds me? What gives me energy, energy not only to do this work but also energy for my own life? From these questions naturally comes the question:

How can I serve my self? If I am not mindful as I give and help and serve, then this is the question that I forget to ask and answer. In the midst of our important work of helping others, it is important to remember our self. In fact, important is an understatement. It is imperative to remember our self. It is our very self that is doing this serving, and without the health of that self, no serving can be done. So how can I serve my self? I believe that in order to answer this question, we must check in with the thinking, feeling, physical, and spiritual aspects of our self. I believe we need to give equal consideration to each of these parts of who we are and ultimately integrate them into a healthy self. If my thinking is dominating and driving me crazy, I want to quiet it. If I am not in touch with my feelings, I want to know them. If my body is crying for rest, I want to sleep. If I have disconnected from my higher power, I want to reestablish conscious contact. By attending to each of these areas, I am learning that the loads I am carrying, usually by my own distorted choices, can be better managed, and I can better manage. Then healthy serving is more likely. It is even more likely if I ask my self:

How can my spirituality serve me? I have found spirituality to be an extremely important area of self, as it is a remarkable source of the energy I was speaking of in earlier lessons on serving. My spirituality feeds me and strengthens me. It helps me to practice the Serenity Prayer, to notice what I can and cannot control. It helps me to control what I can and let go of what I cannot control. My spirituality is a comfort, a companion, a deep well of wisdom, a blanket wrapped around me, holding me close and keeping me safe—safe from others and, especially, safe from me. I call Daisy to "come" many times during the day. Similarly, I want to "come" to my spirituality many times during the day and allow that connection to help me as I help others.

people pleasing

*"I want to
be good."*

Characteristic Described

These next three chapters are interrelated, and yet I have chosen to make them separate chapters because they are each important and distinct aspects of the codependence dynamic. In this chapter, I will be writing about pleasing behaviors— the straightforward desire to make someone else happy or satisfied. In the following chapter, I will discuss being sensitive, a characteristic that can certainly play into our desire to please, and how we respond when we are and are not succeeding at this deep desire to please. The following chapter will look at being adaptable, a behavior that can be useful but can also become an abdication of self in order to try to achieve a number of things, including this pleasing of others.

I know this interconnectedness of these behaviors personally. In fact, I have a lifetime pattern of trying to please others. Either I please them or I don't. I know if I have pleased them, because I am sensitive to their behaviors, expressions, and tones of voice. If I detect that I have not pleased them and/or, even worse, have displeased them or made them angry, then I adjust my self so as to still try to reach the pleasing of the other, which I desire for my sense of well-being.

As we've seen throughout this book, this pattern of mine can be useful and adaptive up to a point, and then it can become pathetic and destructive. The greater my self-awareness about these behaviors and their relationship to one another, the greater my chances for a healthy sense of well-being.

People pleasing is a common characteristic associated with codependence. When I am speaking with someone who identifies as a codependent, it is not unusual for him or her to say, "Oh, I am such a people pleaser." I choose to describe this pleasing behavior as trying to be good, trying to make someone else happy, trying to satisfy someone else, and/or wanting to be liked and thought well of. This desire to please others may involve not acknowledging our own needs so as to make sure we meet the needs of the other person, or going out of our way to keep things under control so that no one is upset. Other dimensions to pleasing behaviors may include trying to make things better for others and trying to avoid conflict.

These descriptors of pleasing behaviors reflect all four of the defining features of codependence as set forth by Dear, Roberts, and Lange and by Dear and Roberts. Pleasing involves a strong case of *external focusing*. In order for me to please you, I need to be paying careful attention to you, your needs, and your reactions. Behind this desire of mine to please you is likely to be my need for your approval of me. I want to be good, to not cause problems, to not have you upset with me. When you are upset with me, I am upset deeply. So I am then more than willing to engage in *self-sacrificing*, to let go of my own needs, if that will help me to help you to be satisfied. *Emotional suppression* can come into action as I neglect not only my needs, but also my feelings, in order to please you and/or to avoid conflict of any kind.

Interpersonal control can also be a factor in our pleasing behaviors. I find this feature of codependence to be a powerful one. Remember, this feature is described as the codependent believing that he or she can fix and control others. In terms of pleasing behaviors, this means that I presume that I have the ability to control the feelings and reactions of others. I am presuming, somewhere in my consciousness, that another person can be pleased, and I know how to do that. I am presuming that I have the ability to keep everyone happy. Pretty presumptuous, huh?

Mary Burch lists "eager to learn and to please" as descriptive characteristics of the border collie's temperament. She elaborates on this in several ways. She speaks about how this desire to learn and to please enables the dog to learn complex tasks. As I wrote in the chapter on "Devoted," the border collie has the ability to be very attentive to the subtlety of its owner's movements, moods, and expressions. This attentiveness, coupled with the dog's desire to want to do what its owner is asking it to do, enable the border collie to work and perform so successfully.

But this desire to please can go too far for the border collie. "Border collies have such an intense desire to please that they can suffer from 'fear of failure.' Dogs who are afraid to make a mistake will either shut down completely or will start engaging in a rapid chain of non-sensical behaviors. This is the border collie's way of saying, 'I haven't got a clue what you want from me so I'll try everything I can think of.'" Burch continues by saying that "Dogs who are trying hard to please may be insecure and in need of consistent praise when they demonstrate desired behaviors."[23]

"Dogs who are trying hard to please may be insecure ..." This makes sense to me. Certainly pleasing others can be an asset, but when we start trying too hard to please, this can either reflect or create an insecure self. In my efforts to please someone else, I may be disconnecting from my self, increasingly focusing on his or her needs and emotions to the neglect of self. Then I, too, may start running around in "non-sensical" ways, trying to get the other person to be pleased or satisfied or to like me, all the while leaving my self behind. The irony of all of this is that I believe these efforts to please others will improve my sense of self, and this may be true to a certain extent if I am successful in my efforts. The problem, though, is that this sense of self and well-being is then dependent on things outside of my self—in this case, dependent on the positive responses I get from others.

For a dog, this can be okay. Though a border collie is smart, attentive, and engaging, its ability to have its own independent sense of self has its limitations. Thus, as Mary Burch explains further about the border collie and pleasing, "When they are paired with an owner who understands the breed and what it takes to work with a dog that is so mentally and physically alert, the relationship can be beautiful." How wonderful!

In the case of us humans, however, I do not want to have an owner on whom I am dependent to please. I do want to please others, to have them like me, to satisfy their needs, but also I want to have the ability within me to know when I am trying too hard, too much, too often to please. I want to attend to pleasing my self as I am trying to please others. I am glad I have the ability to do this. I want to increase my awareness of this and use it.

Though I did say that dogs have limitations in this area of self-development, I do believe that Daisy wants to please me and knows when she has had enough of trying to please me for the time being, and I want to be able to honor that in her as I want to honor that in my self.

Tales Told

As I have told you before, I am Daisy's main person. I guess you could say I am her main owner, to extend the conversation about ownership a bit further. I am the person she literally looks to. Just the other day, Monty was feeding Daisy dinner. He asked her to "sit." I was across the room, and though he was the one offering her food, she was staring at me and not paying attention to him. I walked across the room and stood beside Monty as he continued to say, "Sit," with her food bowl in his hand. Daisy sat for her food as he commanded her, but all the while she stared at me with her big brown eyes and smiling face, which seemed to be gently laughing with love. I am the one Daisy wants to please the most. In fact, if you asked Monty and Grace, they would probably say they have a hard time getting her to even notice them.

Now as I tell you tales about Daisy and pleasing, I am aware that there could be elements of anthropomorphizing her. Mary Burch tells us that the border collie really does want to please, so we know this is true for this breed. The things I am seeing in Daisy as trying to please may or may not be what is going on within her at the time. I have no way to really know. Perhaps in my interpretations of her expressions and behaviors, I am giving human characteristics that are not completely accurate to her experience. Nevertheless, she at least appears to want to please me, and perhaps equally important to this codependent story is that I am pleased by her. Again, I have to say, what a pair we are!

Daisy's overall presentation is one of happiness and pleasure. She often appears to be smiling and laughing. I am not the only one who sees this. A number of people over the years have commented about this to me as they have watched Daisy. She likes to lick the hands and faces of familiar people. When I put my face down to hers, she gives me a lick, which she and I call kissing. I get a Daisy kiss each morning.

To a large extent, though, I believe that Daisy has very particular ways she likes to have physical contact with us, and I believe that in order to please us, she tolerates, up to a point, our wanting more physical contact than she likes. She wants to be a good dog, to keep us happy, so she allows us to brush her for a while, and then she either starts walking away or she makes a soft growl to ask us to stop. In those moments, I believe that Daisy is trying to balance pleasing us with pleasing her self, which has had enough. This same pattern occurs if we are rubbing Daisy with our feet. We first noticed this pattern years ago when we were driving across the United States, with Grace and Daisy traveling together in the backseat of the car. Grace would stretch her legs out and extend them over to Daisy's side of the seat, gently touching Daisy with her feet or maybe trying to tuck her feet in under Daisy. Daisy would tolerate this for a brief while and then softly growl to ask Grace to give her space. Daisy wants to be good, and she wants what she wants, too. Overall, that's a pretty good model of balance in pleasing behaviors.

Daisy is especially pleasing when she allows us to dress her up. We do not do this often. I do not even know when we first put an item of clothing on her, but she tolerates this well. Remember, Daisy has been with us for sixteen years. Grace was eight years old when Daisy first arrived, so Daisy has been a family member through the dress-up years. It makes sense to me, then, as I retrospectively tell this tale of "All Dressed Up," that Daisy was occasionally a party to the trying on of outfits and costumes.

Daisy has two outfits of her own: one is her classic Santa suit for dogs, and the other is an amazing Super-Dog outfit Grace made for her. This Super-Dog outfit includes a cape with a glittered "S," winged goggles, and fancy cuffs. Daisy looks precious in this, and she brings us much pleasure through her cooperation with this costuming and parading around at home. Grace has ultimately gone into fashion design and construction professionally. Her talents in this area were very clear and strong even as she created this special outfit for Daisy when she was a girl. Thanks to her willingness to participate in our silly human amusements, Daisy may in fact possess the first line of clothing designed by Grace Duval.

Daisy has only paraded her Super-Dog outfit around our house, but once she was "All Dressed Up" in her Santa suit in the Lexington Christmas parade. This is another tale about Grace and Amy and their dogs, Daisy and Zeus.

Our Christmas parade in Lexington, Virginia, is just great! Everyone comes out for it. It is usually held in the evening on the first Friday or Saturday of December. Our Main Street is lined with crowds of people watching, and if you are not watching the parade, you are in it. Multiple organizations have floats. Fire and rescue squads from all over the area fill the streets with their lights and sounds. Our schools and colleges have marching units and bands. And our local SPCA always has a group of people walking their dogs in the parade. One year Grace and Amy walked Daisy and Zeus as part of this SPCA celebration.

Daisy was very good about participating in this overstimulating event. She was cooperative and pleasing. Grace put her in her Santa suit, which wraps around her body and has a black belt that holds it in place. The costume also, of course, had a Santa hat that was held in place by elastic under Daisy's chin. Even as I write this now, I am amazed at the notion of even trying to dress a dog up in this outfit, much less parade it for an hour through crowds in a group of dogs it has never met. What we humans think of for our enjoyment! I know the dogs enjoy it too, up to a point, but in thinking about this Santa costume, I believe we were asking a bit too much.

Nevertheless, Daisy and Grace did very well in the parade, as did Amy and Zeus, with walking, stopping, waving, and staying with the special pack of dogs offering their holiday greetings. I was not in the parade, but I followed along on the side and was never so far away that I could not help if needed. By the end of the parade, though, Daisy had clearly had enough of pleasing us. As she and Grace stepped out of the crowd, Daisy started to shake her head and paw at her hat to "get it off!" Her little Santa suit had slipped to the side and was also bothering her, as was apparent by her walking in an awkward way, trying to "get it off!"

Of course we immediately took off her costume. Daisy had done a good job. She was a good dog, and we were proud of her. She had been willing to do what we asked her to do and to do it in a cooperative spirit. She had succeeded in pleasing us and now it was time to stop.

*　*　*　*　*

Would that I had such natural limits in knowing when to stop my self when I am trying to please. Yes, I have made good progress in this area, yet this naturally knowing when to stop can elude me. I believe that my natural state of being is that "I want to be good." I want to please you, to have you like me and think well of me. I have a lot of trouble inside me when I am failing to meet these unrealistic goals. I have my own fears of failure in this area.

I deeply want to be good and cause no problems to anyone. When someone is displeased or disappointed because of me, or I think that person is, that insecurity I spoke of earlier in this chapter comes forward strongly. I then feel unhappy, preoccupied, nervous, and worried. I can go from enjoying my life and feeling pretty sure about what I am doing to wanting to quit everything and live in a cave.

I have to pay close attention to my desire to please others so that I won't be knocked off my center so much that I want to abandon my self and all that is well with me.

This desire to please others runs through my being so much that as Monty and I were recently driving back up to the Adirondacks, I said to him, "I always worry about being a good girl when I'm driving." By this I meant that as I am driving I am concerned about safety, but equally important, I want to please the other drivers around me, not causing them any inconvenience or delays or giving them any reasons to think poorly of me. So, if I am in the passing lane and already driving five miles per hour over the speed limit, and someone is riding my bumper, I may feel badly about holding them up—never mind that the person is being rude and driving dangerously.

As I write these brief tales about me and pleasing, I am telling you that every day I am living small and larger tales entitled "I Want to Be Good"—tales involving everything from how I handle phone calls at work to how I address issues at home to how I conduct my self in public.

To further illustrate the relationship between me and pleasing, I would like to refer back to the tale I told you about me in the chapter on "Smart." As I am writing, I am realizing that the tales I tell in one chapter reflecting the quality I am writing about there are also good tales to illustrate other codependent qualities I write about later. That's how intertwined these codependent behaviors can be. I know it is important for me to write about these characteristics separately so we can have a richer understanding of our self, but at the same time, seeing their interrelationships can give us additional awareness necessary to make healthy changes for our self.

In the tale on my self in "Smart," I had gone to a restaurant in Baltimore, Maryland, with Monty and his good friend. As we settled into our seats and perused the menu, I noticed a table of several women nearby. I decided they had something I didn't and proceeded to feel very insecure and threatened by them. I had no reason to feel this way. This is just what my insecure self did to me in that moment, and, as you know from this tale in "Smart," I abandoned my rational thinking.

I also activated my pleasing behaviors, not in an overt way there in the restaurant, but profoundly within my head. In those brief moments of having dinner out, I decided that I was not pleasing Monty. I decided one of the women in particular was pleasing in ways I am not. As I said in this tale,

> "I wished I was like this woman, this complete stranger
> to us all. I wished I was attractive like her. I wished I
> was so engaging and good company. I wished I could
> be such fun to be with."

I wanted to be pleasing. I believed I was not pleasing enough. I was trying to figure out what would make me more pleasing.

My behavior reminds me of the border collie, which runs around in "non-sensical" ways, trying various behaviors in order to please its owner. Remember, this is the border collie's way of saying, "I haven't got a clue what you want from me so I'll try everything I can think of." That's what I was doing to my self in the restaurant. In my head, I was trying to figure out how to please. I ran from thought to thought, from idea to idea of what Monty might want from me that would please him.

You know how the rest of the tale went. Suffice it to say that my insecure self that decided it wasn't pleasing enough was a real problem, primarily for me, as I ruined my dinner, put an unnecessary dent in my relationship with Monty, and in the end failed completely at pleasing any of us that evening.

Lessons Learned

This is an active, rich area of work for my self, as you have read, and I have learned important lessons that I seriously need to keep practicing in order to develop a healthy relationship with my desire to please others.

Pleasing others can be good. It is fun to cook a meal that someone in particular may enjoy. It is pleasurable to find just the right gift for someone. Satisfying the needs of family and friends rewards us all, and our efforts to bring pleasure to our larger society, in whatever ways we may be interacting with it, can be stimulating and life-changing.

As I please others, I want to stay connected to my self. As I cook meals, buy gifts, or volunteer my time, I want to make sure that I do not lose my self in this process of pleasing. I want to stay in touch with my self in all the ways I speak of: physical, cognitive, emotional, and spiritual. I want to make sure that I am aware of both my internal and external resources for pleasing and that I do not move into neglecting my self on a regular basis in order to please others.

I also want to please my self. As I stay connected with my self, I also want to pay attention to what would make me happy or pleased or satisfied. Those of us who are people pleasers often say that pleasing someone else is what pleases us. I believe this can be true up to a point. I believe, however, that at some point unknown to us, we can cross into feeling mad or fatigued or resentful about all that we have done to please someone else. When this happens to me, it means I have hit my limit on self-neglect in this pleasing process. So why wait until I am resentful or worn out to stop and say, "What about me?" I want to ask my self that question throughout my efforts to please. What about me? What would make me happy as I am trying to make someone else happy? I have also learned that when I ask my self these questions, my answers are not far away. Once I finally do shift into trying to satisfy my self also, I hear my self say things like "I'd like to stay home tonight" or "I really don't want to spend any more money on that."

I want to notice when I am trying too hard to please. It is interesting to me how one lesson learned leads to the next. The examples I just gave about what I might say to my self as I try to please my self and others are really boundaries. To me, this lesson about noticing when I am trying too hard to please is essential to my ability to set healthy boundaries. I want to notice if I am overly focused on others whom I am trying to please. I want to notice if I am preoccupied with how people are reacting to me and my offerings to them. I want to notice if I keep adjusting my needs in order to please them. I want to notice if I am running around in "non-sensical" ways, trying to figure out what I could do that would make them happy. In order to do this, I need to use not only my mindfulness skills, but also the skills of detachment and self-observation, skills that help me to have a bit of space between my self and the other person so I can think and process and act, rather than react.

I want to stop my self when I have made enough efforts to please, whether those efforts have succeeded or not. Being able to do this can be the outcome of my self-noticing I spoke of in the previous lesson. As I am aware of my self when I am trying to please others, I may be taking in information that tells me to let go, to take a break, or to stop. This information may be coming from within me or it may be coming from the other person. Whatever the source of the information, I have learned that stopping my self is important. Yes, this can be challenging as well. If I have succeeded in pleasing the other person, I may want to keep this positive ball rolling. If I have not succeeded in pleasing the other person, I may be driven to keep trying, believing I can figure this out and make him or her be satisfied with me. Either way, I am learning that the greatest chances of real pleasure for all involved come with stopping my efforts to please when I am aware that I have gone too far or am close to doing so.

I don't necessarily know what pleases others. Sometimes other people let me know what they would like, but often I am operating out of what I believe may make them happy. Remember how this is related to a core feature of codependence that says we believe we have the ability to fix and/or to control others. In this case, we believe we have the ability to please others, to know what would please them and to be able to succeed at doing so. It helps me to remember that what I am doing to try please may not be what would please the other person, that what I am doing may be what would please me—though I am not aware of this—and that I had best ask the other person what it is he or she is seeking and then figure out if I have that to offer.

I can't always please others. What they want, I may not be able to offer. What I do offer may not succeed in pleasing them. I cannot be perfect. I cannot always keep all of us happy. Look at all of those superlatives in the previous sentence: *always, all.* Those types of perfect goals can drive me crazy and drive other people away. My overeager self can keep trying to find the right words, the right look, the right expression to elicit the right responses I am seeking to reassure my self of having pleased someone else. In so doing, I am once again running around "non-sensically," and others are often aware of my behaviors as I press in on them, and they either want to go away or want me to go away. I cannot always please others. I want to remember this not with resentment and disappointment, but just as a fact, a lesson learned.

I don't want to be governed by my fears and insecurities. It's my fears and insecurities that can have me trying too hard to please. Just like the insecure border collie trying to figure out what its owner wants, I can be very attentive to the moods, expressions, and behaviors of others. In doing so, I am trying to figure out what would make them okay with me. I do not like how I feel when I am doing this. *Insecure* really is the right word. I feel like I have no solid base under me, no ground on which I stand. And that's because I have stepped off of that ground, which is my own grounding, and into the world of someone else. I'm trying to get into that person's world and adjust it so I have a place in it that feels good to me. When my fears and insecurities arise, I want to be able to notice them, stay with them, and stay on my own turf as I listen to and perhaps choose to attend to the other person. To find a permanent, satisfying place in someone else's world is not real. I want to have my own world that pleases me and that I operate from as I live with and love others.

I need to know what would please me. Often I do not know what would please me. I have not even asked my self. I am operating in an external way, responding to my lists and schedules and other people. I want to regularly ask my self this question as I go through my day: "In light of what I have to do now, what would be a way to please my self as I do that? Or don't do that?" I am finding that the answers are usually not far away, that simply the invitation to my self to consider what would make me happy right now brings forth answers waiting just under my surface, and the answers are often simple ideas that involve stopping, rest, food, exercise, pauses, and silence. Attending to my self in these fundamental ways can bring me much pleasure. Sure, there are many other things that will bring me pleasure as well, but in order to connect with them it is likely that I need to satisfy some of these basic personal pleasures first. Just as Daisy lets us know when she would be pleased by stopping her pleasing of us, I know the importance of my stopping my pleasing behaviors at least long enough to connect with my self and what would please me.

I need to keep learning at a deep level that my sense of well-

being comes from me and my spiritual sources—not from keeping everyone else happy. People pleasing has been one of my ways of operating forever. It is both an asset and a liability. It is a liability when I go too far with pleasing and lose my self in the other person. I want to not only stay connected with my self, but also listen to, soothe, and nurture my self. I want to know that it is as important as anything else to satisfy my needs. I am the only one who can do this. Through people pleasing, I am trying in contorted ways to have others meet these needs within my self. I am learning that this is not possible on a full-time basis. Through my contact with my higher power and with my self, I am able to stay grounded in ways that enable me to cultivate my world and to feel good in it and good about me. Though I have learned that this takes willingness and practice, I have also learned that it is a place of rest and peace and pleasure.

sensitive

• •

*"Please don't be
mad at me."*

Characteristic Described

You can see from the quotation above how "Sensitive" naturally follows "Pleasing." As I try to please, I am extremely aware of what reactions I am getting from the other person, and my feelings can easily get involved in a powerful way.

In this chapter, *sensitive* is defined as being very aware of the feelings and attitudes of others and being easily affected by their feelings and attitudes. This sensitivity can also apply to the way we respond to animals, to music, to reading, to movies—to any of a number of sights and sounds and experiences. Usually if we are sensitive in one area of our lives, we are sensitive in others as well.

In terms of sensitivity and codependence, we find that codependents can be overly sensitive to the feelings of people who are important to them. Because of this sensitivity, codependents strive to avoid open conflict, can be afraid to approach others directly, and respond to someone else's anger by believing it is their fault. Codependents can often feel anxious or worried.

These descriptors create a picture of the internal emotional life of a codependent. Behind all of our serving and pleasing may be a very disturbed emotional center. This is where our sensitivity lives, and this is where a vast array of emotions may be bumping around. Let's look at some of those emotions.

First, I have come to understand that anxiety is often a deeper source of what may be feeding codependence. By anxiety I mean worry and trouble controlling worry. I mean catastrophic thinking and dread. Perhaps this anxiety may involve disturbed sleep, difficulty concentrating, and irritability. Perhaps it may involve extreme self-consciousness and trouble living within your own skin. Any and all of these descriptors characterize anxiety, and I believe they can be an important part of understanding and treating codependence. Seeing codependence as involving an anxious base gives us more ways to help our self to live with our sensitivity and not let it run our lives.

There is also the interactional piece of anxiety and codependence. Even if we are not necessarily wired for anxiety, as codependents we may be living in ways that are causing anxiety, for example, taking care of someone who is sick, juggling more than we can really do, or worrying about having enough money to pay the bills. As the stresses of daily life mount and we take on more and more of them, those same symptoms of anxiety are likely to show up. And, being sensitive people, we are likely to feel them strongly, and they are likely to interfere with our functioning if we do not take care of our self.

In addition to anxiety, our sensitivity may have us feeling some other powerful feelings needing our attention. Fear certainly is one of those feelings. Fear can come from anxiety, but here I want to address it separately. Fear travels with codependence. We are afraid that things will fall apart without our input. We are afraid the other person will get mad. We are afraid the other person will leave us. We are afraid to be on our own. We are afraid to be alone. I could keep writing the list.

These fears can become quite strong and even "terrifying," as someone recently described them to me. These fears are often present and make a difference in our choices and actions. Usually our choices and actions involve our being controlling with the intent, not necessarily known to us, of managing our fears.

I also believe that this sensitive, emotional center is where feelings of shame and guilt can thrive if not attended to. Because the codependent's self of responsibility is so large, it is easy to see how we can feel guilty or ashamed for not taking care of everything just perfectly for everyone. And because we are focused on pleasing others and believe we can, when we have not succeeded at doing so, it is easy to see how we can put that failure on our self. Additionally, others may say things to us that add to our feelings of guilt and shame, and because of our sensitivity, those messages can take root and grow into our sense of self.

There is anger, too. This is such an important emotion to the story of codependence. This tends to be the feeling that we push down the most. After all, how can one succeed at serving and pleasing if one is angry? Wouldn't the other person just go away and confirm all of our fears of abandonment? Wouldn't we look ridiculous and not like the loving, kind person we are known to be? Isn't anger itself the antithesis of self-less codependence? Well, in fact, it is likely to be another one of the deeper bases of codependence. Recently as I was talking with someone about this, I described it as "fossilized anger," meaning anger that is buried and left for a long time, only to surface when we least expect it. But just as with a fossil found, I suggest that we give careful attention to this powerful emotion as it surfaces. And with continued recovery on our part, I suggest that we learn to notice anger and attend to it long before it is fossilized. The Tales and Lessons that follow should help us with this.

Much of this sensitivity that can cause us problems is related to the *emotional suppression* described by Dear, Roberts, and Lange. This defining feature of codependence involves not allowing awareness of our emotions until we are overwhelmed by them. So being sensitive can cause us double trouble if we are not aware, because not only do we easily and strongly feel our emotions, but we push them down or away where they fester and surprise us with their sudden and dramatic appearance. Being sensitive also involves our *external focusing*. Usually we are ignoring our own emotions and feelings to pay attention to those of others. We are focused outside our self and are adjusting our self to the external data we perceive and to which we are attributing meaning. That wonderful, rich emotional center of ours is being ignored, which is the *self-sacrificing* we have also come to know as a defining feature of codependence.

As with the other characteristics I write of in this book, being sensitive is not necessarily a problem. In fact, I believe it is strength. Being sensitive allows me to feel and experience the richness of life. I can be moved by music. I can feel real joy and delight. I can feel excited and loving and grateful. Being sensitive enables me to understand the feelings of my self and others and to respond accordingly. This strength becomes a problem when the feelings I am experiencing start to overwhelm me and interfere with my ability to function and to see my self and my situation accurately.

Mary Burch speaks about this sensitivity in the border collie. As we know, border collies are smart and trainable. Their abilities to be sensitive and responsive to their owners enable them to be such successful workers and performers. But even with the border collie, this sensitivity can become problematic.

"As sensitive dogs, border collies require fair training. They do not respond well to harsh corrections. Border collies have excellent memories and do not forget bad treatment. A dog of this breed can easily be ruined if subjected to harsh training methods. When a border collie creeps along and appears nervous while working, it could be a sign that the training procedures were too tough."[24]

I believe we could say the same thing about the codependent: because of our sensitivity, we do not respond well to harsh criticism, and we can become nervous and practically ruined if we do not manage our sensitivity in healthy ways.

Mary Burch also speaks about the border collie being sensitive to sounds, such as thunder and fireworks. Such loud noises can make them uncomfortable, and they may move to quiet places when these sounds occur. I know that this is one of the ways Daisy's sensitivity expresses itself, and now it prompts my next tales.

Tales Told

As Mary Burch describes this sound sensitivity, she presents a healthy picture of the way the border collie may respond to being uncomfortable: the dog relocates itself to a quiet place. That sounds like a reasonable response to me. My experience with Daisy and her response to sound sensitivity is not always healthy. In fact, there are times when her sensitivity interferes with her functioning and with her accurate perception of her self and the immediate situation.

I don't remember Daisy always having trouble with thunder and lightning, but in recent years it has become clear that those sounds upset her a great deal. Once she becomes aware of the thunder, Daisy's anxiety is activated. She trembles and walks around the house, nervously pacing. She begins to pant heavily and continuously. She cannot be reassured or calmed. Believe me, I have tried.

As a good codependent, I do my best to reassure Daisy that everything is okay, which I know dog experts do not recommend. If the storm happens in the night, I get up with her and move downstairs to where the sounds of the rain and thunder are not as pronounced as they are under the tin roof just over our bedroom. I give her treats to see if that can distract her. No. I make a little pallet on the floor by the sofa for her to rest on. No go. I lie down on the sofa, modeling good resting behavior. She climbs up on the sofa and then on the arms of the sofa, going nowhere but trying to find some place of security, I imagine. But security she cannot find, not the type that will help her to quiet her anxiety and be reasonable about this stormy situation.

Daisy never becomes completely frantic, which I know can happen to some dogs. I have heard stories of dogs breaking through glass doors and running away in response to storms. But Daisy is frantic enough. Her sensitivity has gone mad and her ability to find that secure base is not hers in that moment. It takes a good while for Daisy to finally calm down. Long after the storm has passed, Daisy pants and paces until her adrenaline is diminished and she finally falls asleep, exhausted, I am sure. Then I can fall asleep, too.

Daisy has this sound sensitivity to other things as well. I was aware of her sensitivity to the sounds of guns in the distance, to any surprising, explosive sound, and to a lesser extent to our reactions to her when she is corrected—corrections that are firm but not harsh. This past summer, Daisy added another item to this list of things to which she is overly sensitive: loons. I'll call this tale "Loonacy."

Monty and I were once again camping at Lake Eaton in the Adirondacks of New York. We love setting up our tent near this picturesque lake and enjoying the deep pine forests and blue lakeshores. Daisy and Eddie always get to go on this trip of 600 miles. We keep the dogs on leashes, as is the rule of the state park where we stay. Monty and I were taking Daisy and Eddie for one of our many walks on a path that runs along the lake. It was evening and just lovely. At one point Monty and I both silently noticed a group of three loons swimming out in the lake. We had just turned around in our walk and were headed back toward our campsite. As we walked, we were enjoying the pleasure of seeing the loons and watching their behaviors. Then they started to make their famous calls. For a very brief while, we were able to take in this classic picture and sound of loons on a lake, a special treat indeed. And then Daisy started to notice the sounds of the loons as well, and she became quite disturbed.

With serious focus and a fast pace, Daisy headed toward home with singleness in her purpose: she wanted to get out of there! I had her on her leash, and she would pull on it any chance I gave her. If I had trotted with her to speed up our escape, she would have been pleased. I could tell that Daisy was trembling as she ran. She kept looking back at me as if to say, "Hurry up!"

Daisy had lost her perspective on the whole situation. The loons were not attacking us. They didn't even know we were there. Peacefulness was what the entire environment was about. The colorful sky of a setting sun and the quietness of the pine forest floor that we scurried on were what surrounded us. We were not being chased. We were not being asked to defend or protect ourselves, but Daisy thought we were.

Suffice it to say, we made it back to our campsite without harm. Daisy wanted to get in the car, where she likes to sleep when we are camping. Panting heavily, she drank a bit of water and hopped in the car to calm herself down. Too bad our walk had been cut short, that we could not linger in the loveliness of the evening and the loons. Daisy's sensitivity had succeeded at interfering with her functioning and our outing—nothing major, but unfortunate for sure.

*   *   *   *   *

I have certainly done the same thing to my self, being sensitive as well. I do feel things easily and deeply, and this can be inspiring or this can wear me out. I, too, can ruin a perfectly good time when my sensitivities are in full play.

On the positive side of sensitivity, I believe that most of my life I have been able to feel excited over small things: the anticipation of an outing, a project I may be working on, or a gift I am going to give someone. I can feel pleasure at the way a picture looks on the wall or at the meal I have prepared. I readily enjoy the company of my family and pets and my yard and gardens, which are always calling to me.

I can just as easily feel upset and worried and afraid. I can also feel mad, but I am inclined to go toward the anxious feelings first. I notice people's tones of voice and can be bothered if they seem less than happy. I can watch action/adventure movies sometimes only up to a point, because I start feeling too upset and troubled by what I am watching, even though I know it is only a movie and will likely work out okay. I have a lot of trouble with my feelings when people tell me their sad pet stories, or even when I have to take our pets to the veterinarian, being unnecessarily worried that something is wrong with them and I will find out then.

Recently we had a 5.8 earthquake here in Virginia. I was sitting in my office with a client. I was saying something to him as I started to notice the vibrations coming up through my comfy chair. The vibrations continued as I tried to continue to express my line of thoughts to my client. Finally I stopped and said to him, "This is an earthquake, isn't it?" He nodded and said yes, he believed so. We sat silently for the remainder of the twenty seconds of the quake. We then agreed we should go outside, which we did. Our office complex and parking lot was full of people who had done the same. It was a bit like a party in mood, as no harm had occurred and we had experienced something we don't usually have happen here in Virginia. After a few moments, my client and I agreed we could continue our work and returned to my office. The rest of the day I continued to see clients as scheduled with discussions about the earthquake, but I was not aware of any particular emotional responses from my self about it.

The next morning I woke with noticeable anxiety for no clear reason. I had nothing in my day that was prompting me to be anxious, nor had I gone to bed that way. As the day progressed, though, I realized that it was the earthquake that had set off these feelings of worry and fear that something bad was going to happen. The earth had moved, and I was moved by that shake-up. I am so sensitive that I believe my internal self was literally shaken and moved and activated, and I used my best anxiety treatment techniques on my self as the day went on to quiet and reassure me, to calm my self just as Daisy did in the car after the loon "attack."

Each of these tales shows how sensitivity can interfere with our very basic functioning and how it can keep us from expressing our self accurately and from being realistic in the present moment. I have one more tale about sensitivity that will connect this topic even more directly with codependence.

I'll call this tale "Wait Your Turn!"

Patience is not one of my strengths, though my recovery has helped me greatly with this. I have learned to notice when I am feeling impatient, and I am much better able to manage it and even let it go.

Several years ago I was in a large city with our local dance company. We had been invited to come and perform at a lovely new arts facility in a part of the city that was being revitalized. The building, the stage, and the dance studios within it were truly wonderful. In between rehearsals and performances, I wanted to take a dance class there.

As I was trying to figure out how things worked around that studio, I realized that I needed to use a locker and did not know if they were available to anyone or if they were already rented. I went out into the lobby to ask my question. The front counter was surrounded by people waiting for various types of information and help. I believe some dance classes were just getting out and others were soon to start, so there were a number of people there in that in-between time, taking care of business. And there appeared to be just one person helping everyone.

So I settled into waiting. There was no line. We were all in a small crowd gathered around this counter. The person helping us all was patient and doing her best. I waited. We waited. The help being given took time, and so the "line" did not diminish with any speed at all.

At a certain point, the person at the counter went over to make a copy of something for someone. I decided that would be the moment to insert my question and then get out of everyone's way and back to the dressing room to get ready for class.

"Excuse me," I said, speaking from the center of our little crowd, "I just have a question. Can anyone use the lockers?"

"Yes," she said as she finished making her copy.

I started to move out of the group when a woman behind me said with clear anger, "We all have 'just one question,' and you can wait your turn just like the rest of us!" She was hot, and I was terribly surprised. Everyone around us quieted for those few moments as this exchange happened. I don't remember what I said back to her, as I was so upset. I may have said I was sorry. I may have said something very brief to try to explain my choice of asking the question then. I really don't know.

What I do know is that this exchange affected me deeply for the rest of the day. Someone was angry with me. I had displeased someone, and she had let me know in no uncertain terms. My sensitivity unleashed my worries and fears. I did take the dance class and then went farther into the city to the museums, but all the while I was afraid that I had done something terrible. I was afraid that I had messed up our performing opportunities with this center. I was afraid that I was being reported to someone somewhere. I felt like a very bad girl who had misrepresented my company and my self. I was a guest who did not know how to behave, who was impatient and inconsiderate, and who should be banished!

Yes, that's how far my sensitivity can go. It can cause me to inaccurately perceive my self and my situations. Sure, I guess I should have waited until the counter person looked directly at me and asked how she could help me. If I could not have waited longer, I could have walked away and figured out something else. It is true that I had experienced a collision of my sensitivity and a person who "tells it like it is," but to feel like I should be banished or put in jail for my behavior is just extreme on my part. And it colored the rest of what would have been a happy day for me.

Lessons Learned

I don't want to ruin my good times with excessive fears and sorrows, worries, and anger. I want to feel my feelings, whatever they are, and not allow them to dominate my experiences and my relationships with other people. When my sensitivity leads me to these strongly vulnerable feelings, I am more likely to fall into my codependent behaviors of apologizing for my self, trying too hard to please, or doing extra to make up for being so bad. My sensitivity can also have me running away from people and situations, retreating, hiding, and isolating. My sensitivity can feed my tendencies to act in codependent ways if I do not bring awareness and self-management and spirituality along with me. To this end, I have learned:

Sensitivity can enrich my life. In many ways it is wonderful to be a person who can feel things so fully. I can get excited about very small things, and I can be touched or moved by simple acts. My understanding of feelings enables me to better understand the feelings of others and to respond accordingly. All of this helps me to more fully experience this life I have been given and to live in it in ways that enrich me and my relationships with others.

Sensitivity can ruin my life. Now I know that is a very strong sentence, going so far as to say that my life could be ruined by my sensitivity. Perhaps that is being dramatic and extra-sensitive on my part. What I do know, though, is that smaller experiences can be ruined by my sensitivity, which may over time create a pattern of disruption or erode a relationship. Daisy ruined our evening walk along the lake with the loons. I ruined my good time in a professional dance class. When Daisy and I let our strong emotions take over, we are losing out on some other great experiences that may be going on at the same time that we are falling apart. And those other experiences are also part of our life and our relationships in those moments and are affected by our sensitive reactions and behaviors. I could allow my self to have ruined a dance class, to then quit the dance company, and then to never go back to that big city again. What an unnecessary string of losses.

It is imperative to recognize and allow my feelings. Nothing I am saying about being sensitive is about negating my feelings. One of the core features of codependence is emotional suppression, and good recovery involves learning to allow and express our feelings in ways that are honest, clear, and respectful of both our self and others. That is a pretty tall order, actually.

First I need to be able to notice my feelings and allow them rather than push them down or let them morph into different feelings. Then, as I have learned through mindfulness practices, I want to chaperone my feelings, helping my self to know that I can feel these feelings and be with them without them overpowering me. And then, as I settle my self some by simply being with my feelings, I can understand them better and decide if there is anything else I need to do with them or for them at that time.

It is not okay to let my feelings run away with me. I do not want my feelings to run away with me. It is an awful feeling. It is like being on a runaway horse—out of control, not knowing where this is going or when it will stop. Such runaway feelings can be very damaging as well. Not only do I feel awful and it takes a long time for me to recover from that, but also I damage my relationships with others when my sensitivity-gone-too-far spills onto them. I want to handle my feelings in ways that respect both my self and others. Yelling, pleading, or crawling away does not reflect this respect. Honest "I" statements that are directed at simply representing my self and my feelings are much more on the mark, and I do know it takes work to be so self-assertive. The following lessons can help further with this work.

I want to offer mindful breathing to my vulnerable feelings. Mindful breathing is learning how to be present with my natural breath, feeling the air come into my body through my nose and out through my mouth, noticing the sensations of my breath and allowing those sensations to hold me in the present moment. As I do this, my thoughts become quieter and I become more connected to my self in the present moment. It is here I find that at my core is some peace and quiet and stability. The additional wonderfulness of mindful breathing is that it is available to me at all times for free. I just have to remember to come to this well.

As I strongly feel my feelings, I want to soothe my self and try to put my thoughts and feelings into a realistic perspective. Mindful breathing soothes me. Intentional pauses or stepping away can soothe me as well, and so can getting out of my head and into my body by walking or dancing. What I am trying to do is to acknowledge and identify my feelings and then get enough emotional distance from them that I can see them more clearly and more realistically. I have learned that as my emotions increase in strength, it is likely that my understanding of a situation becomes narrower and narrower and thus not accurate. I am not taking in all of the data, and I am becoming more and more attached to the view I am developing through this narrowing lens. I want to pause and quiet my self, allow my feelings, *and* allow my self to see the fuller picture of the situation. It is likely that both my thoughts and my feelings will be helped by the shifts these steps offer.

I want to address my vulnerable feelings and either do something constructive in response to them or let them go. Allowing my feelings and getting a realistic perspective on the sources of those feelings can be extremely helpful in managing the power of my sensitivity. Beyond these lessons, I have also learned the importance of either doing something in response to my feelings or letting go of whatever has me so stirred up. Sometimes I need to do both. If my feelings are related to the way someone has treated me or to an unhealthy relationship pattern with someone else, I may want to speak with that person about my feelings and offer changes I will be making in order to feel better about my self and our relationship. If I find that my strong feelings are too reactive to a situation and that I did not understand the full picture, then perhaps I need to allow my feelings and then let them go. Similarly, if I have done all I can do to resolve a situation and am powerless to do more, then my emotional health will be greatly helped by accepting my powerlessness. In this acceptance of powerlessness, my feelings have a natural opportunity to soften and loosen their grip on me. This is not to say that I am deciding to accept the unacceptable or to disregard my self. It is simply a path through which I can have more internal peace, a clearer brain, and better options for my self.

I want to continually work on my spiritual recovery, which runs through and can help me with all of these lessons learned. I note that in the previous lessons I spoke of the power of sensitivity. Later in the lessons I wrote about my powerlessness over other people and learning to accept that powerlessness in order to reduce the power of my sensitivity. All of the uses of the word *power* are solid reminders to me of the importance of my spirituality in living with my sensitive self. When I am disconnected from my spirituality, my feelings can run strong and develop a life of their own. They feed on one another, and they develop storylines about my life and other people, which I believe and sometimes will act on with no thought to connecting with my higher power. When I breathe in and out and allow my feelings to flow, I am also allowing my self to reconnect with my higher power. This connection soothes me greatly, steadies me, and supports me. I then can see things I could not see before and open my self to facing many things, including my fears and distress. The irony of this spirituality is that this letting go enables me to have much better control of my sensitivity. Daisy was helped to calm her self by being put in the car after the loon encounter. I want to always remember to help me by putting my self in contact with my higher power.

adaptable

"I want what you want/what you've got."

Characteristic Described

This is a challenging chapter to organize and present. Originally, I wrote a complete chapter on begging. As I have worked with Daisy, me, and my research for this book, I have realized that begging is not a primary characteristic of the border collie or of the codependent, though we do all beg at times. So I thought, "What broader characteristic is begging a part of?" Even that question did not prompt a quick, obvious response from my work. I had to stop and think about this from the continuum model, knowing that I would put begging on the "Going Too Far" end of the continuum. But what would be at the "OK" end of the continuum, and, even more important, what would the title of the continuum be?

After all of this work, I realized that this continuum is about being *adaptable*. In her list of border collie characteristics, Mary Burch includes "adaptable." She also includes "tractable," which I spoke of in the chapter on "Smart." You may remember that *tractable* means capable of being easily led, taught, or controlled and/or easily handled, managed, or wrought. I included that information in the chapter on

"Smart" because those characteristics certainly can contribute to good training and good performance. Those characteristics are also about being adaptable.

Being adaptable means making adjustments to accommodate the needs and demands of particular people and situations. If we are driving somewhere and find that the road we are on is being detoured, we have to adjust our path and likely our time frame and our mood. We make necessary adaptations many times over a day. For example, we had plans to paint a room while the children are at school but one of them is sick and has to stay home; we were going to pay off a particular bill but find that we need a plumber immediately, along with payment in full for their service. These are examples of healthy ways we have to adapt all the time. This has become such a part of my everyday experiences that I often say to my self as I start my day, "I know what I have planned for my day. I wonder what will really happen."

To me this reflects healthy adaptation. This is what is on the "OK" end of the continuum. The strengths of being adaptable include being flexible, being able to negotiate and compromise, and being able to consider multiple needs at once. I love the way Mary Burch describes the gait of the border collie. She says they are "able to suddenly change speed and direction without loss of balance and grace." And as for their body talk, she says the border collie "accommodates quick turns and changes of direction."[25] Changes in direction without loss of grace— that sounds like healthy adapting to me, and that is what I want for my self as life requires this of me.

And being adaptable can go too far. Let's look further down this "Adaptable" continuum.

As we move toward the middle of the continuum, we need to be mindful of not losing our self in our efforts to adjust and compromise. Our healthy adjusting keeps our own needs and feelings in mind as we consider those of others as well, and we make decisions based on all of those factors. When the road is closed, we have to find an alternative route. When the child is sick, we have to change our plans. But further down the continuum, we can become submissive and compliant. We can start letting the needs and feelings of others override our needs and feelings unnecessarily. We can have plans for our day, find that our partner wants us to hang out with him or her, and decide begrudgingly to do what he or she wants to do. Maybe we want to cut our hair but choose not to because someone important to us wants us to have long hair. These types of adaptations start to look like codependence.

Codependents believe that in order to be liked and to get along with people, they need to be what others want them to be. They live too much by the standards of other people. They need to impress people. They pretend to be someone other than who they are. Codependents can have a deep pattern of self-betrayal, apologizing for their self and denying the importance of their own feelings.

I believe that these codependent characteristics relate to many of the qualities I am writing about in this book, and here I am specifically addressing their relationship to being adaptable. When I move from "How can we work this out?" to "I want what you want," I am starting to move into tricky territory for my self. Now I am watching what you want so that I can accommodate that. Maybe I am worried that you will be upset with me if I don't do what I think you want. Maybe I am worried that you will leave me or think I am stupid if I don't. Sure, I have this excellent strength in being able to adapt, but I need to be careful that I am not selling out my self by buying fully into wanting what you want.

We know that dogs will roll over on their backs and ask us to rub their belly. This can be an endearing moment for dog and owner. But part of what is behind this behavior is the dog's submission to the person, the dog's acknowledgment that the owner is the alpha wolf. A more extreme submissive behavior is submissive urination. "Young border collies who are insecure may exhibit submissive urination . . . . In packs, young dogs show that they are submissive to higher ranking dogs by urinating . . . . Understand that a border collie who engages in submissive urination needs some confidence boosting. This is a dog who will benefit from field trips and other new experiences paired with plenty of praise."[26]

This is a clear picture of what can happen to us as we move further down the "Adaptable" continuum. We can become so submissive that we lose our self-confidence and are moving toward losing our very self. An unhealthy humbleness can become active, a humbleness that is apologetic and self-degrading, a humbleness that so deeply feels "I am sorry that I made you mad" that we could pee our pants. This humbleness reflects our loss of power, independence, and self.

And then we can become beggars. Yes, this is how and where I place begging—at this far end of the "Adaptable" continuum. As we started looking at this quality of being adaptable, we saw the importance and value in being flexible and accommodating. As we moved into the middle, I suggested that we moved from "How can we work this out?" to "I want what you want." At this far end of the continuum, I believe we are operating not only out of "I want what you want," but also "I want what you've got." The beggar in me is afraid that I have not yet succeeded in adapting me to you and that I will not get from you what I desperately need—your attention, your admiration, your approval, and your love. I am now riveted on my owner and am ready to perform whatever tricks are needed, regardless of what they may cost my self, in order to get from you what I believe I need in order to feel well and whole. "Please tell me what you need me to do! Please!" I have further lost my power, independence, and self.

In fact, when I think about it, begging is really going off of the charts, off the end of this continuum. We have gone so far in our adapting that we are now engaging in a behavior that is the sure path to the complete loss of self.

I continue to be challenged by describing this continuum, and I found my self in my kitchen talking with Monty about all of this. Being in recovery himself, he pays a great deal of attention to codependence as well. He said about this far end of the continuum, "Ultimate adaptation is total loss of self. You become what you are adapting to." I agree. That's why I said that once we reach begging, we are off the charts, because we are no longer just denying our self, we are now creating a different self that seeks to be and do what the other person wants. And that is exactly one of the ways we describe codependence: codependents believe they need to be what others want them to be. We may mold our self according to the expectations of others or be chameleons, changing our self according to the person we are with at the time.

Begging shows up as we get desperate to know what it is that the other person wants in order for us to get what we want from him or her so we can feel better. As Monty and I talked further, he added, "We have decreasing adaptability by hyperfocusing on this craving of ours." Craving. Great. He used the word *craving*. Begging really can be our craving, our craving for completeness that is dependent on what someone else has. This is why I have already naturally used words such as *desperate* and *lost*. Craving or begging is about self-abdication and total dependence on things outside my self.

Looking at the defining features of codependence as presented by Dear, Roberts, and Lange and by Dear and Roberts, we can see how this "adaptable-gone-too-far" involves a strong case of *external focusing*. I will use their words again, because they so well match what

I am describing: "*External focusing* refers to focusing one's attention on the behaviors, opinion, and expectations of other people and then fitting one's own behavior to those expectations or opinions to obtain approval and esteem.*"[27] Such adapting of self obviously involves *self-sacrificing*. It also involves *emotional suppression*, with the codependent believing that "if I don't ask for what I need or express how I feel, if I adjust my self in this way, then everything will be okay." Further, it reflects *interpersonal control*, the codependent's belief that he or she can fix and control the behaviors of others: "If I adapt enough, I can get the reaction from you that I want."

Tales Told

There are many tales I could tell you about the healthy ways Daisy and I adapt. I have already told you that I have to adapt to external expectations and changes on a daily basis and have learned how to do so not only with ease but even with pleasure as I learn what the day has in store for me. Just recently at Lake Eaton, we had an extremely rainy day, but rainy on and off. Repeatedly I thought I could go to the lake's shore for my morning writing session, and repeatedly I was driven back to camp by the rain, having to let go of sentences and ideas actively in my head and hoping they would be there when I could settle and put them down on paper. I was glad that such disruptions did not ruin my day or spirit.

Daisy certainly has had to adapt to living in our house with us. Necessary expectations have been placed on her as to where she can freely roam, how she is to behave around people, and when she can expect to be fed. She has adapted every time a new pet has joined our family. She is adapting to her aging body. So am I.

---

*"Copyright 2005 from "Validation of the Holyoake Codependency Index," the *Journal of Psychology*, by Greg E. Dear and Clare M. Roberts. Reproduced by permission of Taylor & Francis Group, LLC., http://www.tandfonline.com"

But both of us can move down this "Adaptable" continuum into compliance, submission, and begging, and that's not only where the good stories are, but also from where the lessons come. Begging, especially, takes us right to the heart of where being adaptable can be a problem.

"You are such a beggar," I said to Daisy as we were down by the creek with Eddie on our morning walk. I had just sat on the green bench by the creek to have my minute of watching and listening to the little waterfalls right by the bench while the dogs explore. Instead of enjoying the delights of the morning, Daisy had her nose right on my knee, wagging her tail and hoping for one nugget from me.

I confess I have probably contributed greatly to the creation of this beggar. On our morning walks I always take a little tan canvas bag with dog treats in it. These are treats for "good dogs" as they obey my commands and walk unleashed. We learned to use treats as part of a dog obedience class for Daisy a number of years ago. We had not done so before, but I, in particular, have taken to using treats to train and reward. This type of predictable behavioral conditioning is useful and teaches desirable behaviors. It should not in itself create begging. However, I am very generous with my treat giving, and suffice it to say, Daisy benefits greatly. In that way, I have reinforced Daisy's begging behaviors.

We never feed our dogs from our table, nor do we give them our leftovers or plates to lick. I have agreed with this, as we do not want the dogs to beg. But Daisy's hope springs eternal, and she will commonly sit beside someone at the table eating and stare with her big brown eyes until she is told, "Go away. No beg." Then she reluctantly and slowly moves just a few feet away and pretends that she has turned her head away from us. We have to be firm and clear with her to have her move completely away.

Not long ago my stepdaughter Ava was staying with us, and she and Monty and I were discussing these "I want what you've got" behaviors of Daisy's. We spoke about them in terms of intermittent reinforcement, a powerful behavioral training tool. Intermittent reinforcement means that occasionally and at unpredictable times, the animal or person will receive either a punishment or a reward that has a noticeable negative or positive effect on them. This single event will leave the animal or person anticipating the negative or positive event again. And since they have no idea if or when that may be, they are ever on the alert for it.

So Daisy not only receives her treats at predicable times, such as on walks or when she has followed a particularly challenging command, but also she has been given treats at unpredictable times. Unpredictable times include when food does accidentally drop from the table, when food falls from the counter as it is prepared, or when someone snacking out of a bag spills something on the floor. The speed with which she is on that dropped food is impressive.

I know I have contributed to the unpredictable treats as well. I confess I very occasionally will offer her an extra treat just because I love her, or I will hand her a bite of toast or a cracker. Well, folks, that's all it takes to have her ever loyally following me with her great hopes of something extra-good coming her way. She may miss opportunities to wander while down by the creek or to notice some food already waiting in her bowl because she is so focused on me and what I may have to offer her. In such cases, Daisy is no longer a free agent, living her own little life. She has moved from compliant to craving, and her whining and jumping and nudging tell me so.

*   *   *   *   *

I have brought in this concept of intermittent reinforcement because I believe that it has great power in keeping our codependent behaviors in action, especially our ability to adapt. If I am operating out of "I want what you want" and "I want what you've got," and sometimes I succeed at making these things come true, then I am likely to keep trying these same behaviors. Sometimes I will know what I did to accomplish these goals and sometimes I won't. When I don't know what I did to get the desired response from the other person, I am even more likely to keep trying to decode this situation to get the same or even better results—all of which is taking me further and further from my self.

As my stepdaughter Ava casually said one day after taking care of the dogs, "It's amazing what the word *treats* can do for them." Yes, "treats" can be very powerful. If I randomly receive attention and affection, then I will constantly seek it, not knowing when it will occur again but sure that it will. If someone important to me has said, on even one occasion, that "sometime we should . . . ," I will hold onto that expectation like we have set a date. I call that my "looking for a future orientation," which means that that person is not going to leave me since he or she imagines us doing something together in the future.

Now, these examples could be in a normal zone. It's the extent to which I value them and hold onto them and anticipate them and watch for them that is the unhealthy part of this picture. Some of this reminds me of what I wrote of in the chapter on "Devoted." I have a long personal history of watching people's faces to try to determine their mood and how they are feeling about me. The watching is not just to know these things; it is attached to my begging in my heart for the other person's approval or not being mad with me. The other person does not usually know that this is going on with me, but I sure do. I am overly attached and scanning my environment to externally fill my soul. I think that I desperately need something from that other person.

Perhaps the best way to illustrate all of these dynamics— adapting, begging, intermittent reinforcement, and loss of self—is to revisit the tale I told you about me in "Devoted"—once again, a tale told to illustrate how one codependent behavior can richly illustrate other codependent behaviors because they are so interrelated. They merit separate chapters, and they merit revisiting through other lenses.

In the tale, after our dinner I asked Monty to wash the dishes before the next morning. Monty did not like my request, and I knew it. This prompted an argument between us, and then our pattern set in of Monty withdrawing and me becoming anxious. As the tale went, I proceeded to try to calm my self by several walks down our country driveway while trying to figure out what would make things okay between us again, returning each time to our living room where Monty was watching television in the dark. I would try to speak with him in friendly ways to reestablish our relationship so that my abandonment fears would be quieted. The first time I tried this, I was not satisfied with Monty's response to me and went back out on another walk. The second time I returned to the house, I succeeded in engaging Monty enough to be reassured that he was not going to up and leave me that night.

This tale was written about being devoted and what can happen if our devotion starts slipping down the continuum toward "Going Too Far." It highlights our watching and attending behaviors as well as fears of abandonment. But even as I wrote this tale for "Devoted," I was aware of the adjusting behavior I also was telling you about as the story went on. In fact, as I wrote it, I was struck by the ridiculousness of the adapting I was doing over dishes—but not really over dishes, as I clarify. Washing the dishes, the simple request/task of washing the dishes, got lost in my attachments and fears. "I want what you've got" became my guiding light.

Here is what I wrote in "Devoted":

"Most of all, I can be compelled to abandon me so you will not abandon me. If I am not taking care of my self in such moments, I will let go of whatever I want, need, think, or care about just so you will come back to me. Never mind the dishes that I wanted to have washed. I'll gladly change the subject and fix popcorn if that reestablishes the fine balance I need to feel secure and reassured that the object of my devotion is not going away. I'll watch you carefully and obsessively until I am satisfied that you are okay with me, forgetting to consider if I am okay with me."

What a beggar I had become in this story. My begging was probably not overt, but it sure was alive inside me. I was adapting my self moment by moment in order to reduce my anxiety and restore the relationship as I needed it to be. As I say above, I'll let go of my request for the dishes to be washed if that will make things okay. I will be friendly and not demanding if that will make things okay. Never mind my reasonable request. Never mind my feelings about ways we share responsibilities in this house. Never mind me. Each time I "never mind," I am adjusting and moving down this "Adaptable" continuum from adapting to submissive to begging. I am giving away my strength and self-respect and personal grounding, and soon thereafter I may well, once again, have lost my self. I may have you, but I have lost me. On a Saturday night in our television-lit living room, my adapting may bring me some relief and reassurance, but in the long run this adapting does not serve me well.

I have one more tale about Daisy and begging as I move us to some Lessons Learned about all of this adapting.

At Christmas, all of our animals have their own Christmas

stockings hung on the chimney, which runs through our living room. Some Christmases we have as many as five or six pet stockings hung. I could swear Daisy remembers Christmas and her stocking. On Christmas morning, as we follow our family tradition of very long gift opening, Daisy waits patiently for hours as we carry on. Then, when we move to the chimney stockings for the pets, she becomes her sweet, animated self, jumping and jumping and, of course, begging for someone to help her get her stocking down and unwrap her special package of—appropriately named—Beggin' Strips.

Daisy has Beggin' Strips, and I have beggin' strips. We both know what we like and want. We both pursue it actively. And we both can carry it too far. When I get so caught up in "I want what you want," and especially "I want what you've got," such that I will do, say, or be almost anything I believe the other person wants from me, then my codependence is in full swing and merits my recovery. If I am jumping and jumping, eagerly trying to get someone else's love, attention, and approval, there is no way I am connected with my own love, attention, and approval.

Lessons Learned

Being adaptable is a strength. We know that being rigid and stubborn can cause us problems and leave us stuck. Flexibility enables us to make necessary changes with balance and grace, just as the border collie was described early in this chapter. Getting all upset about something that has changed and that I have no control over is a waste of my time, energy, and good spirit. I want to be able to adjust and move on with minimal to no damage.

I do not want this strength to become my weakness. In my willingness and ability to be flexible and resilient, I do not want to adjust to the level where I have given away my strength and my self in the process.

Adapting becomes a weakness if in the doing I let go of my self. In my recovery I have come to know and understand that my ability to connect with and operate out of my healthy self is what keeps me from losing my self in others. In this case, my connection with my self helps me to not lose my self as I adapt, because if and when I do lose this self-connection, I have lost my strength and serenity. Someone recently said to me, "I had contorted my self in so many ways [to adapt to her living situation] that there was no real me left." In this process, she had become both physically and emotionally sick, and, ironically, her adaptation did not yield the results she was trying to achieve. Actually, this is not uncommon. In her pursuit of "I want what you want" and "I want what you've got," she received conflict, lies, and betrayal.

Healthy adaptation involves consideration of both self and people/situations outside of our self. The key word in this sentence is "both." It is important for me to be able to listen to and consider things other people say to me, suggest, and/or request. It is equally important that I then listen to my self about what they have said and pay careful attention to what I think and how I feel about it—how my physical self is reacting to what was said and what my spirit is telling me. I need to take time to do all of this before I make a decision to change or adjust. Maybe I even need to step aside and give my self some extra time to fully hear my self and to make a decision about how to perhaps accommodate what is being asked of me. It is this fuller process that enables my healthy adaptation. It involves consideration of both my self and the other person, and it shows respect for both my self and the other person. Self-respect yields respect from others and supports successful compromising and negotiating.

Submission and compliance can be tricky and require that I really connect with my self before submitting or being compliant. Sometimes I do need to submit or be compliant. When I was under the age of eighteen, I had to submit to requests from my parents in order for us all to get along and in order to live in safe and healthy ways. In workplace settings, each of us has times and situations where we have to submit or comply. Often there is no compromising with deadlines or "the way things run around here." Whether we like the rules and requirements or not, if we choose to work there, we have to work within the structures given. But submission and compliance can be tricky. As I make decisions to bend in the ways being asked of me, I want to make sure that at a deep level this is really okay with me, that I will not be violating my self in ways that make me physically and/or emotionally sick. I want to know that I can live with my self if I make this decision to adapt in this particular way. Can I still be true enough to my self as I accommodate you? Can I live with my self if I adjust to what you want?

"**No beg.**" I do not want to move farther down this continuum into being so attached to "I want what you want" and "I want what you've got" that I beg. We say "no beg" to Daisy, and I must also say it to my self. Begging is unbecoming and unproductive. It puts me in a powerless position where I am leaving it to someone else to give me what I want. And they may or may not do so. And further:

I am a lovely and loving person who does not need to beg. Begging is bound to be about lack of self-confidence, self-respect, self-trust, and self-love. I could go on and on. It is so clearly about the lack of self. My continuing assignment is to develop my sense of self, to return my focus from the external to the internal, and then to grow out from there. The very nature of codependence is this looking outside of our self, and so I know that the essence of my recovery involves this development of my lovely self.

I do not want to be a victim of intermittent reinforcement. I do not want occasional good things to be enough for me. I do not want to be ever hopeful that one particular nice, reassuring thing will happen again, even though it hasn't for years. I do not want to be watching and waiting and hoping that today is the day that "treat" will show up again. Such watching, waiting, and hoping leave me completely vulnerable and dependent on things outside my self.

Begging highlights the external orientation of codependence. Begging is clearly about looking outside my self for what I want. It involves believing that I can be filled by people, things, and situations external to me. And the more I move down that continuum from healthy adapting to begging, the more external I become in my focus and the more attached I become to "I want what you've got."

Unhealthy attachments to "I want what you've got" can produce unbecoming behaviors on my part. These behaviors may include repeating my self, following someone around to try to continue a conversation, trying to force a conversation, trying to force an answer, seeking reassurance, asking too many questions. Among the less obvious behaviors may be eavesdropping, watching from a distance, or offering gifts and money. I am mindful not to slip further down that line of sneaking and peeking, but the begging can have enough power to encourage those types of behaviors as well.

An external orientation is not only misdirected and unattractive, but it also deprives me of developing my internal self. How in the world am I going to get to know and take care of my self if my focus is somewhere else? When I am busy watching someone else's behaviors and responses, I am likely not watching mine. When I am busy contorting my self so as to get something from them, I am likely not evaluating how I am doing and whether my choices and behaviors are best for me.

I need to be aware of when my adapting is shifting toward self-abdication. *Abdication* is a strong word, and I wasn't sure I wanted to use it here. I looked it up and decided it is indeed what I am saying. Abdication is about the giving up of sovereign power, relinquishment of the throne. Self-abdication came to me naturally as I was writing this lesson, because I do mean that I want to be mindful to not move to full and complete relinquishment of my own power and strength. So as I am traveling down this "Adaptable" continuum, initially making necessary adjustments in what I can and will accept or do, I want to be aware within my self of when I start to feel unsure about my choices and the behavioral changes I am taking on. These internal messages are important cues to me that I need to stop and carefully examine what I am doing and likely turn around and head back toward healthy adaptation. I need to be aware of when I am letting go of listening to my self. This is the crucial point at which I intervene on my own behalf and can restore a more balanced response to whatever adjusting I am doing. If I miss this important moment, submission, compliance, and begging can become the next stops on this train to loss of self.

Self-development strengthens my ability to adapt in healthy ways. The more I know and trust about my self, the stronger I will be in the face of requests for me to adapt. This knowing involves my commitment to stay in touch with my self and my abilities to listen to my feelings and needs from all of the areas of self: physical, cognitive, emotional, and spiritual. In doing these things, I know that I will be developing my self-confidence, self-respect, self-trust, and self-love— all of which are important in and of themselves and will help me to figure out whether I want to make a change in my direction with balance and grace or not make the change at all.

Self-development quiets my submission and begging and soothes my soul. This is the really good news in all of this: we can

possess the unwavering concentration required to gain control over a belligerent ewe using only the border collie eye."[29] This "eye" is an intense, convincing look, almost like a stare, that border collies use to move and control those sheep in their lives.

Some of these border collie features that contribute to their herding abilities make me smile as I think of us codependents. My experience with codependence is that I, too, seem to have strength and endurance. It is as though my body is built to keep on working and producing. I can work well independently, and I can also get very focused and intense in trying to make something happen. I bet there are even times when I use the border collie "eye" to nudge some point of mine or request of mine along. In terms of herding itself, my strength and focus can go toward trying to pull everyone together for an assortment of reasons.

I have noticed that when I am in a group setting, I often scan to see what everyone is doing and how they are doing. If we are socializing, I don't want to miss a thing. If we are working, I want to make sure everyone is doing what I think they should be doing. There are times when I catch my self operating out of a belief that "everybody does everything together." And not only do I want everyone to do everything together, but I want everyone to do everything together *now* according to how *I* think it should be done.

Recently I was in a work situation where four of us were operating as a team toward an agreed-upon common goal. Suffice it to say, our work went very well, with an excellent outcome that met our goal. Afterward, I was speaking with my husband about the project and realized some of the herding-type behaviors I had been experiencing while working with this team. When there were lulls in our activity, I would look around to see what everyone else was doing, to make sure they were doing what I thought they should be doing. If they were playing around or having fun for a few moments, I could feel annoyed, believing they were wasting our time and making us unproductive. As I told Monty about these thoughts and behaviors of mine, I realized how active my codependence was at those times. I wanted to control what everyone was doing so we could accomplish this goal that I was so attached to. In an effort to humorously modify this obsessiveness, I found my self saying, "So what if everybody's off task!" and "God forbid there be a lull!"

Yes, heaven help us if there is a lull! What a border collie-type thing to say. I operate out of constant activity and engagement. Let's keep going. If we're done with this, let's move on to that. Just like the border collie running around to herd, I, too, run around great distances in seemingly endless activity. Traveling with all of this activity is an emotional aspect to herding—excitement. Not only do codependents and border collies share the physical and mental capabilities for herding, but we also share some of the emotional draw of that activity. "Give the border collie a chance to interact with some livestock and watch the excitement begin!"[30] Give the codependent an assignment and watch the excitement begin. We, too, can get caught up in our purposefulness and put our whole heart and soul into making it happen, striving to engage and activate others along our way. In fact, codependents report that they can feel bored or empty if they don't have a problem to focus on, just as the border collie feels bored if he or she doesn't have a job to do. We all need and feed on engagement and excitement.

Herding involves several of the defining features of codependence as set forth by Dear, Roberts, and Lange. By its very nature, it involves *external focusing*. We are focused on things outside of our self, in this case in order to get the job of herding done. In part, this tendency toward *external focusing* is as natural to us as it is to the border collie. We also engage in this *external focusing* in order to ultimately gain approval and esteem. This may not be completely clear to us as we strive to pull everyone together to accomplish some goal we have in mind, but in fact our sense of self becomes dependent on our ability to make this happen.

As we live in this world of *external focusing, self-sacrificing* can naturally follow. Codependents' deep beliefs that they should place the needs of others ahead of their own and that it is their responsibility to devote their energies to solving the problems of others leave them vulnerable to this disconnection from self. Herding invites this self-sacrificing as codependents narrow their focus to the multiple tasks at hand that can lead to their desired outcome for all. With their chins lowered to the ground and their gaze fixed on their herd, codependents can easily start losing track of other relationships and responsibilities and their own feelings and needs.

Herding is really all about *interpersonal control*. Herding involves controlling the livestock, being able to pull all together for health, safety, and practicality. Codependents believe we have similar abilities to fix and control others, and we operate out of that belief system without much awareness that that is behind what we say or do. But it is true. We have a deep desire to keep things under control or to keep a handle on situations. This is hard enough when we are dealing with just one other person; when we are trying to manage and control multiple people at a time, we are further challenged and can get further lost from our self. Codependents believe that without our effort and attention, everything will fall apart. In actuality, it may or may not fall apart, but what my recovery has taught me is that with such intense external and narrowed focus and such imposition of my self on others, *I* will surely fall apart.

Tales Told

As you know, Daisy has no sheep to herd. She does have us humans and the other creatures that live with us, especially cats. In the chapter on "Hardworking" I told you about the jobs Daisy takes on here at our home: providing companionship, greeting, and protecting. She also takes on herding as best as she can considering the variables of her life. It has been easy for me to see this herding behavior in her over the years even though she tends no livestock.

First, I must mention again the physical capabilities for herding that Daisy shows us. Perhaps one of the best places we see these features in full swing is when we are at a beach. Daisy has traveled with us to many beaches. She has run on the Atlantic and Pacific beaches and has walked, played, and run on the beaches of all five of the Great Lakes. She has been a lucky dog to travel with us, and we have been lucky to travel with her. Daisy gets to run on these beaches when the laws allow and when no one else is around, and boy, can she kick up her heels, cut tight corners, and run like the wind!

Such was the case once when we were camping at Huntington Beach, South Carolina, one of our favorite places, which you will be hearing more about in later tales. Monty, Grace, and I were hanging out on the beach under our umbrella, reading and resting and watching the ocean. We were in an area where we could be alone and Daisy could be free. Occasionally beachcombers would walk by, visit a bit perhaps, and then move on. Then we noticed two people riding bicycles close to the water's edge, traveling north up the beach. Attached to each bicycle was a tall, flexible post that was attached to a long leash, at the end of which was a border collie. Two border collies were running along with their biking owners and having a wonderful time. Daisy ran out to speak to them, and the owners circled back to us to inquire about Daisy. They were professional border collie breeders and trainers and were struck by her excellent style and athleticism. Her great display of herding behaviors on the beach drew their attention, and they wanted to know more about her. Nothing much else came from this. We enjoyed sharing stories about border collies, and we went by their campsite to see the agility course they had there for their dogs. I guess this tale is really about Daisy's validation as a border collie, with true form and endurance and agility and obvious abilities to do what border collies do: herd. It was nice to know that the border collie experts were impressed with Daisy. It helped us to know Daisy better, too.

But in her simpler existence here without sheep or a truly rigorous border collie life, Daisy is left to herd other pets and humans. When a new pet comes to our house, Daisy can become very focused on it. In fact, she can be persistent in trying to get into a room to see an animal that may be there for its safety. For example, Grace has had two pet rats over the years, and Daisy consistently wanted to push her way through the door and go to the cage to get to know them up close. Three cats have joined our family over these years of Daisy's life with us, and each time she greets them with nose nudges, licking, and occasionally the lowered-to-the-ground border collie posture, trying to move them from one place to another. To this day, as Daisy is in her sixteenth year, when she and Eddie are outside running, Daisy cuts him off and insists upon outrunning him, even if he has a head start.

What first drew my attention to Daisy as a herder, though, was how she positions herself in our house. Daisy will sit or lie in two particular places that are central to her being able to know what is going on with each of us when we are scattered throughout the house. For many years, one of these places was on a step halfway upstairs. From this vantage point, Daisy is positioned between the bedroom/computer room upstairs and Grace's room at the foot of the stairs. She can also look through the stair railings into the living room, where she can see and hear additional action. Further, from Daisy's step, she can look out the window of our front door at the base of the stairway and see what is happening outside. Even as Daisy more slowly goes down these steps these days, she often pauses halfway down to look out the window of the front door. I've always imagined that Daisy loves her step because this is the best she can do with her abilities to herd us all together. She is able to monitor each of us and move herself through the house according to our activities and movements. And she does that. As we all move to other rooms and collect in particular places in the house, more than likely Daisy is right there with us, especially if we are all together.

Daisy's other herding location is in our dining room on the rug at a spot where she can see directly into the kitchen from one angle and directly into the living room from another angle. She has used this spot for years. Granted, she is in our way as we move back and forth through these rooms, but she persists in being there, again, I imagine, because she can know what in the world is going on with her herd of humans and respond in responsible border collie ways.

*   *   *   *   *

You see, I, too, can position my self around my house in ways to know what everyone else is doing. This is where I noticed early on these herding similarities between Daisy and me. Most of the time when I am home, I am readily and easily engaged in my own activities, paying attention to what I want to be doing and doing just that. But sometimes I am preoccupied with what others are doing as well. This may be because I think I know what they should be doing, or I am worried because we are upset with each other. In these cases, I can slip into my herding behaviors. I have a variety of ways that I herd, some obvious to others and some not. Either way, the examples of my herding involve unbecoming behaviors on my part that have me paying attention to someone else's business when it is no business of my own. These unbecoming behaviors may include following others around the house or yard, watching from a distance to know where they are and what they are doing, and/or monitoring their progress or lack thereof on a job I think should be done. I may make comments to herd them in the direction I believe they should be going, or I may adjust my own hopes and plans so as to put this herd together in the way I believe it should be and in the way that lowers my anxiety and helps me to feel that everything is under control. After all, that's what herding is about: getting everyone/everything under control.

And with a different motivation but similar herding drive, I can act in these ways when I am having a party at my house. Whereas my herding can be motivated by wanting things my way or by not wanting someone to be mad with me, when I am entertaining my herding is motivated by wanting everyone to have everything they could possibly need to have the most wonderful time. I am sure I am not alone with this desire, but I hope all are not as overwhelmed as I can be during the event with my efforts to herd everyone to the time of their life.

I am going to tell you a party tale—"The Border Collie/ Codependent Entertain"—but first here is the thread of the story leading up to my tale.

As I started writing this book several years ago, Monty asked me, "So are sheep alcoholics?" If codependents are the border collies, it does make sense that the sheep are alcoholics. From a nonrecovery point of view, here's how that looks: We border collies believe that if we don't herd the alcoholics, they will wander away and get into trouble of some sort. They may run into coyotes or wolves, or they may get lost. We believe we need to put them in place and protect them from all sorts of things. We also believe that we need to herd them simply to do everyday tasks and responsibilities. In the sheep world this would be the basic act of the border collie moving the sheep from the shelter to grass and back to the shelter.

With this metaphor in place, I was further entertained when I read a story in Mary Burch's *The Border Collie*, working with the same border collie/sheep relationship issues.

> "There is a cartoon that shows a group of sheep standing on their hind legs at a crowded cocktail party. The sheep are holding their drink glasses and they all look terribly bored. One of the sheep notices a border collie coming in the door and says, 'Thank goodness! The border collie is here . . . now the party can start!'"[31]

In this case, Mary Burch is particularly commenting on the excitement the border collie brings to herding. I think it is also amazing that this cartoon places the border collie in relationship to sheep having cocktails and the neediness of the sheep for the border collie to come in and do what the border collie does—in this case, run around and herd them all up with energy and excitement.

Well, that's exactly how I can be when I am the border collie at my own party. When I was thinking about a tale to tell you about me and herding, at first I was satisfied with what I have already told you about how I act in my home under some circumstances and in social situations. Then I realized that both the internal and external picture of me as I am entertaining really is like a border collie in a field full of sheep.

As you know, we live on a river in Virginia. One of the things we love to do on the river is go tubing. Just in case you don't know what this is, it is the simple sport of filling a large inner tube from a truck

party is ahead of me, the border collie hostess. Will they know where to get off the river? Will they know how to get up to our house? Will they be hungry and start looking for food? Will they get into the food without my supervision?

I should have stayed behind or gotten off the river first so the potluck part is set up just right.

I bet everyone is waiting for me and doesn't have a clue what to do until I can get there.

Herding Up Dinner

I want only these foods to be put out for snacks first.

I want these foods on these plates so they look just right.

I want everyone to wait until all of the snacks are out before they start nibbling.

People asking me,

> *Where should I change my clothes?*
>
> *Where should I hang my wet clothes?*
>
> *Do you have some extra dry clothes for me?*
>
> *Have you seen my _____?*
>
> *Can I use your oven? How do you set the oven temperature?*
>
> *Where are your spices? Do you have any fresh herbs in your garden?*
>
> *Can the dogs be loose in the yard?*
>
> *So-and-so needs directions to your house for dinner.*

How can I coordinate all of these dishes for dinner so that they arrive at the table at the same time, looking and tasting great?

How are these other guests who were not on the river with us but have joined us for dinner? I need to give them some special time.

And where is so-and-so? I thought she was coming to join us for dinner, too.

Do we have enough plates? Utensils? Serving utensils? Drinks?

Does anyone need help getting their food? Finding a place to sit?

Does everyone have someone to talk to and feel welcome and connected?

Herding as the Evening Goes On

Did everyone enjoy the birthday cakes and ice cream?

Did all the Leos get recognized? Do they feel included and considered?

Is everyone okay? What can I do for you?

What is everyone doing now? What am I missing?

Should we light the campfire?

Maybe we should go back down to the river.

Maybe we should all stay in the front yard.

How can I keep everyone together? What would please them? Do they want a fire? Music? More food?

What will keep people here at the party? What will make them want to stay here in one place so that I am reassured that they have had a most exciting and amazing time?

What a glimpse into my border collie being when I feel so responsible for my herd! I do enjoy our Leo Fest, but that is pretty surprising considering the strong and persistent herding instincts that are in operation for me and could easily overwhelm me and the delights of such a fun party at my home. Gratefully, I have learned some lessons that help me to moderate my herding thoughts and behaviors so that I do not completely lose track of the pleasures of the present moment or the presence of my self in that moment.

Lessons Learned

Herding can serve an important purpose. Certainly in the animal world, being able to pull a herd together is important for safety and survival. The herding the border collie does so naturally is enormously useful to the shepherd and the sheep in terms of not only safety and security, but also utility and practicality for the business of raising sheep or other livestock. Sometimes herding is also important for us humans. Fire drills and other types of evacuations are orderly ways of moving large groups of humans to safety. In amusement parks, museums, and other tourist-type places, we are herded as a group from one event to the next to bring order, information, and pleasantness to our time there. Schoolchildren are herded from the classrooms to the cafeterias and bathrooms, and when we are driving our car into a construction area, we are herded into the designated detour. Each of these examples presents herding as helping to create necessary order and safety for those involved. It is when herding is not about these essential purposes that it can become more of a problem.

I am not a shepherd. No one has asked me to tend and to lead everyone. I do have family members whom I have some responsibilities toward, but even with them I try not to herd them in the direction I think they should go unless it involves safety, security, and survival When I start trying to herd people because I want to have things go my way or because I am trying to keep a handle on a situation much bigger than me, this is where I believe that my herding instincts are going too far. There could be the most spectacular fireworks in the world going on outside at the party I am giving, and yet if some of my guests prefer to remain inside for whatever reasons, I must not try to herd them to the fireworks display. If I have been trying for a long time to get my entire family together for a week at the beach and one of the family members does not want to come, I cannot make him or her join the herd.

People do not need to be herded. With the obvious exceptions presented in the first lesson, people generally do not need to be herded. People are able to think for themselves. They are able to listen, to problem solve, and to take action in the ways they determine are best for them. I can offer them information and ideas, but then I need to see them as capable and willing to function as responsible adults with minds of their own and leave them alone—no nudging or border collie eye.

People don't like to be herded. Have you ever noticed someone pushing back against you when they detect you are trying to move him or her in a particular direction? I don't necessarily mean move him or her physically. I also mean trying to make that person change his or her mind, beliefs, or plans. Our developmental goal as human beings is to grow into competent, independent adults. When we are treating others like they are not, we are offending them and infantilizing them. They get the message that we know what is best for them and are insisting upon it. This is disrespectful and demoralizing to them, and frustrating and self-defeating for us.

People cannot be herded. Most of us have heard the analogy about trying to herd cats. Someone may be describing a situation where he or she was trying to get a group of people to come together in some way, and in speaking of unsuccessful efforts to do so, says, "It was like trying to herd cats." Well, that's my experience as well. People cannot be herded. Even in evacuations, there are people who stay behind, and even when we are stopped in our car in a construction area waiting to go on the detour, occasionally there is someone who insists upon using the emergency lane to speed past us all. The codependent in me can forget that I cannot control the behaviors of others. In my enthusiasm for what I want to share with others, or in my extreme measures to keep everyone happy all of the time, I can step in and try to move us all in the same direction—a direction I am prescribing. In those moments, I have forgotten that I do not have such control over others.

My herding behaviors can be unbecoming. This I said in my tales, and it bears repeating again here as its own lesson. As I lose my self in trying to "move us all in the same direction," I may not only nudge and use the border collie eye, but I also may behave in a number of other indirect and deceitful ways. Manipulating, lying, guilt-tripping, sneaking, peeking, following, and/or telling half-truths can come forward and into action as ways to make things happen the way I think they should. The border collie does not do these things. The border collie is clear and direct and firm. If I need to herd, I want to be this way. If I don't need to herd, I want to be able to recognize this and certainly not engage in behaviors that are so deceptive and destructive to my soul.

My herding behaviors disconnect me from my self. Yes, herding involves serious external focus. It is all about watching things outside of our self in a focused way and trying to impose our will on whatever our focus is on at that time. In this case, we are talking about narrowing our focus onto others and moving them as we believe is best for them. As I engage in this external focus, I become more and more preoccupied with things outside my self and lose my connection with my self. If I am not careful, the only remaining connection with my self is my driven belief that I need to make such-and-such happen for all of us. I have disconnected from my centered self, which notices my broader thoughts, feelings, body, and spirit and which, in that noticing, is able to respond to my self in an honest and respectful way.

I can offer/suggest/direct and then stop. In *Disentangle: When You've Lost Your Self in Someone Else,* I wrote an entire section on setting healthy boundaries,[32] and I believe that this lesson is about doing just that. It is okay and even important for me to offer whatever it is that I have to offer to a person or situation—food, money, ideas, opinions, help, information—and to even give specific suggestions or directions about how to obtain, use, maintain, or spend whatever it is that I am offering. And then it is equally important for me to know when to stop, and to stop. At my own Leo Fest, I can wish we were all traveling in our tubes down the river together, but to insist that we do that is obnoxious and impossible. I can want everyone to gather around the campfire, but to go and interrupt conversations and other activities to make everyone come to the fire is also obnoxious and impossible. I must know how and when to stop my self, and leave others alone to enjoy themselves as they wish.

I can only do my part/it is important that I do my part. In my herding, with enthusiasm and energy for getting others to do what I want them to do, it is oh-too-easy for me to not be doing what I am supposed to be doing. This is the other side of the previous lesson: I stop trying to make others do something, and I make sure I am doing whatever it is that I have control over. I love the way we can apply the Serenity Prayer to our recovery from codependence. The Serenity Prayer invites us to accept the things we cannot change, to change the things we can, and to know the difference between those things we can and cannot change. In codependence, I find that I am often trying to control what I cannot control (other people), and am not controlling what I can (me). Returning my focus to my self and what I do have control over in any and every moment is my point of strength and peace. Being able to settle my self in my tube and enjoy the person there with me, and to feel the water and see the beautiful scenery we are passing through, is a much healthier place for me than looking ahead and behind and wishing for something different than what I already have. It is from this position of personal strength that I can then see, know, and do my part—which perhaps in that next moment is to navigate my self safely through a tricky rapid.

Herding my self to health is really my job. This sentence has several important words in it. First, the words *herding my self to health* convey the general message that I want to shift my herding behaviors from others to my self. I want to remember how good I feel when I am applying the Serenity Prayer and allowing that application to help me work with the things I can control. The health I can gain from doing this is not only emotional, but also physical. When I am running around trying to micromanage others so as to achieve my desired end, my body is not being attended to, and I can get worn down and sick. Additionally, I am likely ignoring my spiritual health as I take on the herd in a godlike way. The word *really* in this lesson is a strong reminder to my self that I have not been given the job of herding others; I "really" have been given the job of herding my self. That brings me to the words *my job,* which is the next empowering reminder that I am responsible for my self and for the task and pleasure of my own care.

I can be as difficult as a belligerent ewe when herding my self. All of these lessons can be easier said than done. I can get something in my head about how I want things and people to be. I can justify my ideas in a variety of ways. I can convince my self that I should keep nudging and trying to corral us all into some amazing place or experience. I must be disciplined with my self when I start moving into this herding of others and redirect my efforts to managing and controlling my self. That belligerent ewe has her heels dug in and is resisting. I can be the same way as I try to work many of these lessons. In these moments I must come back to my self and remember how bad I feel when I am exhausted and frustrated from herding and how good I feel when I do my part and leave others to do their own.

I need to keep working on doing my part and then "going with the flow." When I was describing what tubing is, I noticed that the third action on the list was "going with the flow." In that case I meant the flow of the river, but as I wrote those familiar words, I thought how ironic it was to suggest that I was going with the flow at our Leo Fest when in fact I was herding as hard and as fast as I could without being an obviously controlling hostess. I imagine everyone on the river at the Leo Fest was having a fine time without all the tweaks and input I wanted to add. They were going with the flow. I trust that unless someone asks me directly for help or information or direction, that person doesn't need me to offer those things. Especially through my spiritual growth, I am able to allow people and things to be as they are, not as I believe and insist they should be, with everyone all herded together, safe, well, and happy. When I apply these lessons to this desire Daisy and I share for a well-herded world, I can let go of things outside my control and enjoy the ride a whole lot more.

reactive

"Woof! Woof!
What's going on?"

Characteristic Described

In *Disentangle: When You've Lost Your Self in Someone Else*, I write about learning to act, not react.[33] This idea appears in the section on "Detaching," which is about learning ways to get emotional distance so we can think and see and decide how we want to respond to a person or situation—not react to them. In looking at the meanings of *react* in the dictionary, I note that *reactive* is defined as responding readily to a stimulus. The dictionary also notes that *reactivity* can mean having a response that is resistant and oppositional to the stimulus that provokes the reaction. Either way, whether our reaction is too quick and/or whether it is in direct opposition to what is coming our way, I maintain that I want to learn skills that enable me to move from being reactive to being able to respond from my centered self.

My experience with my codependence is that my healthy excitement, alertness, and responsiveness can move too quickly into radical reactivity. In my twelve-step fellowship, we sometimes describe our selves as "making molehills out of mountains." I have come to understand and appreciate this. This is saying we can minimize problems and the ways we are treated in order to keep things under control and peaceful. I agree. I also believe, though, that we can do what the original saying expresses—"make mountains out of molehills." I know that I can take things too seriously, and in doing so I can make more out of a comment or action than was intended. Then I can react abruptly, dishonestly, dramatically, and with damage to my self and the other person(s). My focus has become narrow and fixed, and I am barking way too much.

Being reactive can be seen as a particular extension of being sensitive. Certainly, our sensitivities to the feelings and reactions of others make us vulnerable to overreacting. Our sensitivities to wanting to please, wanting to avoid conflict, and wanting to manage our fears and anxieties have us primed to react if and when we determine that these fundamental desires of ours are being thwarted and/or our efforts to achieve them are failing. So although reactivity can come from being sensitive, I believe it is an important behavior in and of itself for us to examine and learn from. Being reactive can be an immediate loss of self. What we say or do as we react may well not be what is true for us. The things we say and do then may hurt us and leave us in a more vulnerable and self-defeated position than ever.

Being reactive is also about being in extremes: *always, never, forget it, hopeless, give up, never change, can't, won't.* As you know, I believe each of those words can have an appropriate time and place in our lives in which they are true. I am not throwing them out. I am saying, though, that if they are our common reactions, then we are keeping our lives and our selves limited and shut down. Once again we are seeing that it is the extremes of codependent behaviors that become problems, not the behaviors themselves when they are moderated and centered. In this case, centered responding is healthy; reactivity grounded in extremes is a problem.

Considering these extremes involved in reactivity, let's look further at how this relates to codependency. Some of the words that come up in the literature describing codependence readily reflect extremes: *empty, overly sensitive, any lengths, my fault, inadequate, worthless.* Operating out of an all-or-nothing mind-set contributes greatly to these extremes in self-assessment and the way codependents experience their world: "I have failed if I haven't pleased everyone." "My work was wasted if everyone wasn't 100 percent enthusiastic about it." These can be unexamined reactions that come out of our sensitivities and jump immediately to the extremes.

Being reactive certainly involves *external focusing.* When I am reactive, I am usually responding to something outside my self and likely to something that may be keeping me from getting the approval and esteem that I am seeking from these outside sources. "The codependent is seeking to fill underlying needs for approval and belonging. This is a normal aspect of social interaction. The defining features of codependency that fed into the theme of external focus refer to an excessive and abnormal reliance on others' approval and acceptance.... It is this excessiveness that distinguishes the codependent characteristic of external focusing from the normal human need to monitor and attend to others' opinions and expectations."[34]

Reactivity also involves *self-sacrificing* in a couple of ways. First, Dear, Roberts, and Lange describe this behavior as neglecting one's own needs for those of others, and just as with *external focusing,* they say that this normal behavior becomes a problem when there is "a socially abnormal degree of effort being directed to meeting the needs of others."[35] Again, we see where extremes are causing the problems, and I believe our being extreme is part of being reactive. *Self-sacrificing* is also involved in reactivity in that it can be a total loss of self. Our reactions have disconnected us from our own needs and feelings and left us vulnerable: "Fine! Then I quit!"

Interpersonal control means that we believe that we can fix and control others. I believe that much reactivity comes from us when those beliefs are challenged, such as when we are in a situation that is obviously not in our control. Our reactions in such a situation are about that loss of control we thought we had or want to have, and they may be misdirected attempts to gain control over that out-of-control situation and/or to regain the control we thought we had in the first place.

Emotional suppression is an important aspect to being reactive as well in that it is defined as not allowing or not knowing one's own feelings until they are overwhelming. This is exactly what feeds reactivity. When I become overwhelmed, I react. Whether this is because I have taken on too much or have pushed my feelings down and out, I can reach my breaking point—with or without advance notice—and my reactivity ignites. What an unfortunate thing to do to my self and to others. What an unfair way to abdicate my healthy self who is available to me and has important things to say to me if I will listen.

In terms of the border collie, Mary Burch never uses the word *reactive* to describe this breed, but she does offer examples that reflect both healthy and unhealthy demonstrations of this behavior. Certainly border collies' abilities to listen to and to respond to the commands of their handlers show healthy responsiveness. Through this responsiveness, border collies are able to perform the tasks they love to do, and their handlers accomplish the tasks they intend to do. Border collies' sensitivities to the gestures and moods of their owners also can be examples of healthy responsiveness, with the dog taking actions or making adjustments in response to what its owner wants. But we already know from the chapter on "Devoted" that this type of watching and reacting can go too far. The dog can misinterpret signals and overreact to signals, for example, in Mary Burch's story, causing the dog to be disqualified from a competition.

Mary Burch does use the word *neurotic* on occasion in her book. *Neurotic* means that there is a mental or an emotional disturbance within the individual that does not affect his or her entire personality, but that does cause specific and noticeable physical and psychological reactions. There, I said it: reactions. Neurosis does not *have* to be about reacting, but it *can* be about reacting—overreacting, actually. Mary Burch's dog, Laddie, was overreacting to mailboxes. There is no reason to react to mailboxes, except when we may be receiving an important piece of mail. Mary Burch and I have both already told you about the border collie's oversensitivity to loud sounds such as thunder and fireworks, which can result in strong reactivity on their part as well. And though Mary Burch offers a healthy description of the border collie as "sensibly reserved toward strangers and therefore . . . an excellent watch dog,"[36] I have told you how Daisy completely overreacts to strangers and men in hats and how difficult this has been to train out of her. This invites some more tales about Daisy and me and our being reactive.

Tales Told

One night I was lying in bed just about to fall asleep. My husband was working nights, and our daughter was off at college. All of a sudden I heard some rumbling in the distance that alarmed me and brought me immediately back to my awake state. Note that in the process I did not stir at all.

Just a fraction of a second later, Daisy, who was asleep on her mattress on the floor beside me, jumped up and went into frantic barking. She ran over to the window and barked and then went out into the hall and onto the stairs, where she continued to bark in earnest.

Of course, I jumped up to see what terrible thing was befalling us here in the dark of midnight. Had hoodlums driven down our country driveway, and were they now approaching our house with guns? Had the wood stove in the living room exploded and set the first floor ablaze? Or was our chimney on fire, with flames bursting from it and the neighbors coming to alert us?

There was nothing to be alarmed about.

I looked around quickly and thoroughly, then I reassured Daisy and my self, and we both lay back down. What we had probably heard was a distant train. In addition to living by the river, we live by a train track that follows the river. After my living here twenty-six years, you would think I would have the sounds down pat and have no cause for alarm. But no; both Daisy and I carry a propensity for hypervigilance and overreacting.

As for Daisy, part of this is in her breed, and I like it. I've said that if Daisy is asleep at night, I can sleep, because I know there is no harm within a ten-mile radius. She is a good watchdog.

But she overdoes it.

As you know, we have never been able to train Daisy out of barking as our family and friends arrive at our house. And heaven help us all if the person arriving has on a hat or some peculiarity of dress. She can be unrelenting in her barking at them upon their arrival, and almost defiant of our efforts to stop her, until we have to spray her with the water bottle.

Daisy jumps from nothing to all. She can be lying asleep in front of the wood stove and in a second be up and barking as if we are under attack. If we are at the beach, she reacts the same way when other dogs and their owners walk by. And in a hotel room, any bump or sound from outside our room has her immediately up and on duty.

Daisy's on-duty work never goes beyond barking. She

does not lunge or bite at anyone. This would not have been okay with us. She just persistently and frantically barks until her sense of danger has passed.

*　*　*　*　*

I, too, can overreact. Carrying some anxiety in my self, I can too easily catastrophize if I am not careful. Calls and messages from attorneys worry me until I can return them, because I think I've done something wrong. The smell of smoke in our house immediately sets off my concerns about a house fire. When people say they need to talk to me, I fear there is a problem or they are mad with me.

I can even overreact to Daisy. One morning Daisy and I were waking up. As she tried to stand up from her bed, I saw that she was falling over. Her right leg was not working. She was holding it up in an unusual way and could not put it down on the floor. She tried to stand a couple of times and could not get up. I was immediately distraught. What happened to Daisy while she slept? Had she had a stroke? Oh, no! What to do? My adrenaline was pumping, and I had catastrophic thoughts right away. I stooped down to her to do I don't know what— probably to hug and reassure her, to calm us both down so as to get a handle on this situation. It was then that I noticed that one of her claws was caught in one of the rings on her collar. I freed her claw, Daisy stood up, and we continued our day as usual. What a reactive explosion for me upon awakening! What a way to start my day!

Just recently, I again overreacted to Daisy. I had come home from a long day at work. Daisy was traveling through the house with me in her manner of greeting when I noticed that she did not want to use her back left leg. She kept flicking that leg and throwing it off to the side as she tried to use it. She was clearly bothered by this leg, and her efforts to use it created an unusual presentation. All of this was also interfering with her ability to walk, as she would almost fall over and would just stop and flick that leg. Of course, I reacted strongly. I was immediately afraid that something very bad had happened or was happening to Daisy. As in the last tale, I was afraid that she had had a stroke and that I was seeing neurological damage. I called my husband to the scene. He calmly suggested that perhaps something was in her paw. We laid her down on the dining room floor, and I took her left back leg in my hands to examine it. There, between two of her paw pads, was a noticeable-sized stone. I removed it, Daisy hopped up, and she resumed her running and jumping greeting of me. I was extremely relieved and grateful. I was also sorry that yet again I had put my self through such strong reactions. I suggested to Monty that we then take Daisy and Eddie out for a walk, saying Daisy probably could use the walk. What we really knew was that Nancy, the other border collie, was the one who really needed the walk.

All of this overreacting throws me off center and out of my self. It puts me into some extreme state, and I lose my serenity and my sleep. It sets off my anxiety, with all the related activation of my adrenal system, and then wears me out.

Once again my codependent posture, which ever has me on the alert to the external, has taken over, and I abandon my good reason and healthy self for yet another trip into frantic excitement— excitement I swear I don't like, yet I keep coming back for.

Lessons Learned

A drive down to Myrtle Beach several years ago helped me to see the progress I have made in managing my tendency to overreact.

I called this trip a "special mission" because its intent was to get our then-eighteen-year-old daughter to the US Marine Corps Ball.

In so doing I was able to get my self to my private, oceanfront "writer's retreat" to once again get a jump start on this book.

We left Richmond, Virginia, at 5 a.m. as Grace had requested, with me picking her up at the front door of her college dorm. My husband had warned me repeatedly that we would be driving into bad weather—that a severe front would be passing through the East Coast as we drove south. He told me to watch for heavy rains, strong winds, and the possibility of tornadoes. Tornadoes associated with this system had already caused damage in Alabama and Mississippi.

I drove on I-95 for the first hour and a half with Grace, who had had only three hours of sleep, sound asleep in the passenger seat. The rain must have started around 6:15 a.m., with big drops but nothing else. Then, around 6:30 a.m., while we were driving in North Carolina, my internal alarms started going off about this situation. I passed an exit with many well-lit stores and gas stations. The second I passed it, I could see even in the predawn light that we were driving into an extremely dark and low cloud formation. All of my alarms came into play, with fear and catastrophic thinking. I woke Grace gently with my voice and touch, asking her to be awake with me and be a second set of eyes as we ploughed through nearly zero-visibility rain on this notoriously busy and dangerous interstate highway.

I turned on the radio and found the nearest public radio station, which was indeed issuing tornado warnings. I did not know the names of the counties under watch and warning relative to where we were. I wanted to get off the highway and to center us in safety. I badly wanted to get off, but that would be nearly thirty minutes in coming, as traffic was very slow and the exit was far away.

I could continue to tell this traveling story in detail, describing how I chose to handle this weather and driving situation until about 11 a.m. that day, when the severe weather warnings expired. But I won't, as my real mission here is to process with you the lessons I have learned about overreacting and how I applied them in this storm.

I will tell you the ending, though, as that is what gave me an additional perspective on my lessons learned. Grace and I got to Myrtle Beach just fine. We had left early enough that we were able to be close to being on schedule for each of our destinations.

After Grace left me at the condo, I took a sweet, deep nap on the sofa, with the ocean sounds pouring through the door as the storm cleared the coast and continued to move out to sea. When I woke, I turned on the weather channel to learn that four tornadoes had touched down in North Carolina. One of the tornadoes had been deadly, killing eight people. The people had been warned at 6:29 a.m., and the tornado hit at 6:38 a.m. It had been just east of I-95, about 100 miles south of where we were at that same time.

What I have learned is:

My reactions can hurt me. When I allow my self to be lost in another person or in a situation through my reactions, I am disconnecting from important internal data and abilities that can help me with the situation at hand. I can no longer know my true thoughts and feelings, and I may act in ways that are counterproductive to what I truly need, desire, or mean. I am placing my self in an increasingly vulnerable position and simultaneously diminishing the resources available to me.

My reactions can hurt others. I can say and/or do things that are destructive to their sense of self and that they may remember for a very long time. I can say things I don't mean to say, tell things I never intended to tell, or issue ultimatums I did not even know were about to come out of my mouth. In my hyperadrenalized state, I can convey my fears and anxieties unnecessarily onto others, disabling us all.

There will always be things out of my control. Since some of my reactivity comes in response to things out of my control, I will again state the importance of actively living the Serenity Prayer: sorting what I can and cannot control, acting on what I can control, and deeply learning ways to let go of what I cannot control. It may take my frustrations and/or failures to realize I am trying to control something that is not mine to control. The important lesson here for me, though, is that when I do recognize something as being out of my control, I need to deeply and honestly believe that and adjust my self accordingly. Driving through tornado territory certainly offered a situation that demanded my active sorting of what was in and out of my control and how to respond, not react, accordingly.

Reasonable responses from me are welcomed. Remembering that I am looking at all of these behaviors on a continuum, it is important to say that my reasonable responses will be welcomed, if not by everyone, at least by me. I will have thoughts and feelings about things, and I will want to express them in ways that respect my self and the other person. I may disagree. I may be unhappy. I may be afraid. I may feel strongly about something. It is important for my mental health that I recognize these parts of me and express them in ways that are true and clear, not overwhelming and destructive.

I cannot afford to lose my self in my alarm. I have not been able to rid my self of my fears and worries, but I have learned that I can manage them and thus create for my self more successful outcomes. I can think. I can make decisions. I can pause and center my self. And that is exactly what I did for Grace and me as we traveled through the storm. I got us off the interstate three times that morning, losing nearly two hours of traveling time, but proceeding only as I felt ready and safe. I was able to do that because I have also learned that:

Mindfulness returns me to my center and allows me to notice important data about my self and my environment. As I proceeded down I-95, I kept returning my focus to my breath and to the sensations within me and around me. By so doing, I was able, for the most part, to have a stable center from which to operate. Even when I was challenged by sleepy Grace about this not being such a big deal and "Why are we worried about tornado warnings? We never pay attention to them," I was able to not react to her, but rather act from my own sense of me and the situation.

Going from nothing to all is not useful. There is a lot in the middle. Overreacting can mean that I was feeling just fine and now I'm all upset. Let's think of a light switch versus a dimmer switch. The light switch is either on or off, dark or light. The dimmer switch allows a progression from dark to light and vice versa. That's what I want for my thinking and feeling self—to be able to keep appropriate gradations of each as I move through a situation. Codependents are known to be all-or-nothing in many of our behaviors, and so it can be with our emotional self, too. It is up to me to adjust my dimmer switch as I notice I am losing my self.

I personalize too much. This is not necessarily about me. Codependence seems selfless. It seems as though in our focus on others, we have no self. Ironically, much of what drives codependence is a self-centeredness directed at protecting the undefined self we do and don't know. So when there is conflict, disagreement, or trouble, we take it personally. A lot of overreacting is bound to happen if I take things personally, for example, if I think someone is not joining me for dinner because he or she doesn't like me, or if my husband is unhappy and I think it's my fault. Even weather conditions can be personalized: "This storm is happening because I shouldn't be making this trip." The world does not revolve around me. Things are what they are. People do what they do. It's likely it doesn't have anything to do with me.

I don't need so much excitement. It has also been said about codependents that we like excitement—good or bad will do. Excitement must help us to feel alive. Overreacting creates lots of excitement, and I have learned that that excitement can go on for days, depending on what happened. I no longer want that intensity of feeling. I have come to know serenity and am quite fond of it. Oh, I experience peaks of all sorts of excitement still, but even in the midst of those storms, I'm already ready for the peace of a centering nap by the ocean.

tenacious
••••••••••••••••••••••••••

*"I know you want
me to stop, but I
don't want to."*

Characteristic Described

This chapter was first entitled "Determined." I liked the word and the concept, and I did some writing about being determined. But I realized as I further studied my self and the border collie that "Tenacious" is actually the quality that captures the aspects of codependence that involve "I know you want me to stop, but I don't want to."

In a side box listing seven characteristics of border collies, Mary Burch includes "tenacious." I knew what it meant and didn't. So I looked it up in the dictionary: "not easily pulled apart . . . persistent in maintaining or adhering to something valued or habitual."* I like each of these definitions. "Not easily pulled apart" speaks for itself. If I am working, I don't want to stop. If I am trying to find just the right gift for someone, I don't want to stop. I don't want to be pulled away from these things. And then there is the word *persistent*, which again speaks to holding onto something or somebody, especially if, as the definition

*By permission. From *Merriam-Webster's Collegiate® Dictionary*, 11th Edition ©2012 by Merriam-Webster, Incorporated (www.Merriam-Webster.com).

says, we are holding on because of habit or because it means a great deal to us. Other words that describe *tenacious* include *tough, strong,* and *cohesive.* Note already how each of these words can be a positive attribute. Being tough and strong, and even sticking with someone or something, can be a beautiful human characteristic that enriches our lives. But we can go too far in these behaviors. Our tenacity can become sticky and problematic in a number of ways.

Sometime in the recent past, Grace was telling me about a specific grant proposal she was working on for a wearable arts event. She was in college and had become quite accomplished at finding, submitting to, and getting funded for the various wearable art shows that interested her. In this particular case, Grace had to repeatedly make calls and send emails in order to get her submission done in time. She had followed up on every contact she was given, politely and persistently asking her questions and making her funding requests until she succeeded at getting what she wanted. In responding to her story, I said, "Grace, you certainly are tenacious, and I admire that." To which she responded, "Well, guess who I learned that from!"

I laughed and thought about it. We have been very close over the years, and she has seen me a number of times really pursue what I wanted, whether it was an item in a store, an answer from someone, or a project I wanted to complete. I am sure she has also seen me pursue conversations that went too far and work that could have waited until the next day.

Yes, codependence can involve tenacity, and it can all begin at a healthy place. The codependent is often operating from an energized self that brings alertness, responsiveness, and excitement to much of what we do. We start off feeling really interested in and inspired by whatever it is that has caught our attention. We may even become determined in our pursuits. This determination, however, may lead to our being controlling, which can lead to our being rigid and compulsive. That's how this quality can go too far.

That's a lot of words to throw at you so fast, and yet that's how our tenacity can progress. Our desire to do something can move from reasonable efforts to our wanting to control everything in order for that to be accomplished. We want things to happen in the ways we have prescribed, and we won't stop until we are satisfied—that's the compulsive part.

Being tenacious relates to earlier chapters on "Hardworking," "Adaptable," and "Reactive." Working hard does involve my staying with the job at hand in order to be able to accomplish my assignments, and my determination can help me to be successful in my work, and, as we have learned, it can go too far. Being tenacious can certainly invite being adaptable. If I am in deep pursuit of something or somebody, I am likely to be willing to adapt in various ways in order to achieve the goal I have set for my self. My tenacity is the undercurrent of my efforts to get what I want and, if necessary, to sacrifice self through adapting in order to do so. And being reactive also can have my tenacity as its source. When I am reactive, it may be coming from my efforts to control people, places, or things I have no control over, and my reactions, though they may be unhealthy and misdirected, are coming from the part of me that is after something and doesn't want to let it go.

All of this is to say that once again, the qualities I write about in these separate chapters interrelate in many ways. Seeing their relationships to one another is important, and examining them separately can help us tremendously in our recovery. Such is the case here with being tenacious. When we are able to know and to see this quality in action within our self, our ability to intervene on our own behalf will be greatly helped if we are willing.

Yes, if we are willing. This topic of being tenacious is really about our unhealthy attachments. By unhealthy attachments I mean our holding onto people and/or things when doing so is hurting us, causing us problems with our health and our lives. We don't want to let go! We are not willing to let go. This is where being controlling, rigid, and compulsive comes into play.

Looking at various ways codependence is described, I am struck by the terminology that speaks about these extremes in pursuit: preoccupied, focused to the point of neglecting self and other responsibilities, more than your fair share, devote your energies completely, no matter what happens, work hard enough, and do things yourself in order for them to be done right.

Being tenacious certainly involves *external focusing*. I am not only paying attention to something outside of my self, but I can become overly focused and preoccupied with that external object of my attention. I can become obsessed with someone else and lose sight of practically anything else. Then, I am unhealthily attached.

This unhealthy attachment easily leads to *self-sacrificing*. When I become so focused on someone else, I am bound to be neglecting my self and other responsibilities. If I am so willing to give my complete self to someone else, there will be no energy left over for my needs. If I am determined to drop everything I am doing so that I can do for others, I will never be able to do for me. Ironically, my tenacious pursuit of what I have decided I want is taking me further and further from my connection with my true self. I have abandoned even my self-awareness.

And *interpersonal control*, which describes the codependent as having an entrenched belief in his or her ability to fix and control others, must really feed tenacity. If I am operating out of this belief about my abilities, I will only be encouraged to keep trying to do whatever it is that I have decided must be done. I will pursue and pursue, acting out what Dear and Roberts say about the codependent: "[C]ontrolling is clearly a core component of codependency . . . a strong need to control other people and situations."[37] So again the extremes come into play, with codependents not only tenaciously holding onto this belief, but also tenaciously holding onto their behaviors of going to any measures and/or taking over completely in order to get what they believe they want.

These descriptions of codependents and tenacity are mirrored in what Mary Burch tells us about the border collie. "Most border collies are intense dogs who can become absolutely focused on a task. These dogs possess the unwavering concentration required to gain control over a belligerent ewe using only the border collie eye. . . ."[38] There are those words again: *intense, absolutely focused, unwavering concentration,* and *to gain control.* It just so happens that this is exactly what the border collie is supposed to do. It is in its breed and training. As Mary Burch tells us, "endurance is [its] trademark."[39] So bravo, border collie! The border collie knows what it is to do and does it with calculated tenacity.

Codependents may well have this tenacity in our breed and training as well, but often we are pursuing work/tasks/people (sheep) when no one has asked us to do so. Unlike the border collie that has been assigned these jobs requiring such focus and bringing things under control, we have not been given such assignments. And even if we have been asked to do so, if we are not mindful, we will fall into "I know you want me to stop, but I don't want to" as we lose track of our self in pursuit of the goal laid out there.

The border collie, on the other hand, is trained when to stop. Mary Burch has a lovely way of describing this:

"When a border collie completes a herding job, the shepherd indicates that the job is done by saying,

'That'll do.' When a border collie dies, his shepherd will frequently bury him on the hillside with his sheep, marking the grave of his faithful helper by carving the dog's name on a stone. Beneath the dog's name, some shepherds also include the final command, 'That'll do.'"[40]

"That'll do." What a lovely sentence. It suggests a job well done and a stopping point for that job. I think I would like to adopt that sentence for my personal training. A few tales below will help you see why I say this.

Tales Told

Six years ago in the spring, Monty, Grace, and I were camping at Huntington Beach, South Carolina, one of our favorite places to go. Daisy and Eddie were traveling with us as well. While we were sleeping in tents at our camp, Daisy and Eddie were comfortably sleeping in the car. We do not allow them on our furniture at home, so Monty says they love to get to stay in the car because this is as close as they get to sleeping on a sofa.

One beautiful morning, Grace and I had a spontaneous work session on this book, consulting about the book's content and her photography of Daisy and me. We sat in our lawn chairs at our tent site talking, laughing, and getting excited again about this project, which as you know had been underway for many years even at that point.

Shortly thereafter, Monty, Grace, and I, along with Daisy and Eddie, headed down to the beach for our morning walk. I was sure I had decided on the next essay I would write, probably on herding. I felt clear on general examples I wanted to use and trusted my spirit to say even more about tales and lessons.

And then things changed.

We were walking on the nearly abandoned beach having a swell time, Grace totally into photographer mode, running around the beach in her gypsy skirt, taking photos from as many angles as she could muster of Daisy and me. Because we were the only creatures anywhere near, we let the dogs run free of their leashes. We were having a fine time.

I decided I should have a red top on for the photos instead of the green I was wearing. This would show off black-and-white Daisy better and possibly work with the cover design we had been discussing. Grace had on a red sweater. So we decided to switch sweaters. Monty circled back around to join in our craziness and to laugh at Grace, who now had a winter scarf on with a tank top while I was buttoning up her red sweater on my body, two sizes bigger than hers. In this moment of joy together, we lost track of the dogs.

Eddie had seen a couple of dogs entering the beach over the dunes and took off toward them. Daisy followed suit, and would have gone first had she been the first one to see them. No amount of calling them stopped them. Monty whistled at them. I ran wildly toward them, trying to intercept them before they reached the other dogs. They ignored us and ran on, determined to do what *they* wanted to do: meet the other dogs.

And they did. They got there first, much to the surprise of the other dogs' owners and to our chagrin. No blood was spilled; nothing bad happened except the chaotic flurry of activity that can occur when dogs and owners unfamiliar with each other come together.

I felt terrible about the whole incident. We removed and leashed our dogs. As Monty and Grace took Daisy and Eddie away, I went back up to the other owners and asked, "Do you need anything else from us?" They had checked their dogs and curtly said, "No, things seem to be okay." I paused in case they had more to say, and they did not. I walked down to the shoreline and joined my rattled and stunned family. We walked back down the beach to our tent site, dogs leashed, us dazed.

The rest of my day was profoundly affected emotionally. My pleasing and sensitive qualities came into full play. The dogs had behaved poorly, and I had been irresponsible. My anxious, catastrophic thinking was active. The situation had been out of my control and should not have been. Forget writing. I was too agitated, worried, afraid, and ashamed. What would I have to say that would be meaningful? I could not do that until I knew what was meaningful for me in all of this.

The next day I was still working my way out of this emotional abyss. I was still not sure what I had to say about this incident. I thought of writing about fear, which had become dominant for me the previous day. I was afraid our dogs might have hurt the other dogs. I was afraid the dog warden would be called and at any point they would show up at our campsite and take Daisy and Eddie away from us. Then I looked at my book outline and realized that part of what got us in trouble the day before was Daisy and Eddie's tenacity, tenacity that overrode their training, their obedience, their loyalty, and any good sense. They were possessed, in a split second, by what they had laid their eyes and their hearts on, and they were not to be persuaded otherwise. Being tenacious, they ignored the familiar people, voices, and kindnesses they know. In a heartbeat they were attached and gone.

Daisy has always kept a small part of her hardheaded, determined self. We have never been able to train or reason it out of her, though she has attended dog obedience classes. When we tell her, "Everything's okay, there's no need to bark," she will continue. When she sees another dog and we say, "Stop and stay," she may eventually follow our command, but it is after our persistence and with her great reluctance.

Daisy has a certain presentation when she becomes consumed by determination. In fact, she looks like the border collie Mary Burch describes with her absolute focus, her unwavering concentration, and her border collie eye and posture. Her focus is pronounced. She is looking only at what has caught her attention. Her head is protruded a bit forward, and her eyes are riveted on whatever she sees or hears. We try to interrupt her gaze so as to break this powerful attachment. She resists. We turn her head toward us. She pulls it back. Her body is rigid and attentive, somewhat crouching, preparing to move, perhaps with great vigor, toward the object of her attachment.

And this is what can get this good dog in trouble.

*   *   *   *   *

I am struck by how the word *attachment* has naturally emerged as I write about being tenacious. Being focused and determined can be important and useful. We establish plans and goals, and it is our determination that helps us to reach our end desires. Being determined helps us to figure out things that puzzle us, things we want to create, or things we want to know and understand. Again, it is back to considering these codependent qualities on a continuum. To a certain point, being tenacious is valuable and productive . . . to a certain point.

Tenacity can be carried to an extreme and result in unhealthy attachments. Some of the original writers on codependence remind us that codependent behaviors in their more extreme forms involve a relinquishment of self and an obsession with others, an obsession that is fed by tenacity and that melds the obsession into compulsion and destructive attachments.

Frankly, I know this progression well, as it lives in me in small and large ways.

In small ways, on a daily basis, being tenacious helps me and hurts me. I am so determined in running my own business to complete X, Y, and Z before I leave each day that I don't get home until 9 or 10 p.m. My tenacity adds to my being the "Last One Home in Rockbridge County." All is quiet on the streets as I leave, and I meet few cars as I drive the fourteen miles to our river home, a home I love and from which I am often absent. This is sometimes not good for me or my family.

I can be determined to finish something before I or we can go somewhere. I can be determined to have things just as I wish for a party or special occasion. I can be determined to figure out something that has caught my attention or to resolve a disagreement before I can go much further.

None of these behaviors is necessarily a problem unless, as the *Diagnostic and Statistical Manual of Mental Disorders –IV* states, they cause us problems with social or occupational functioning.[41] So what does that mean? Does my being tenacious inconvenience others? Does my being tenacious offend others or hurt others? Does my being tenacious inconvenience or hurt me? Am I exhausted by my schedule? Have I put aside too many other things to do whatever it was I was determined to do? Have I become frustrated, anxious, depressed, compulsive?

In larger ways I have been tenacious in my efforts to make unhealthy relationships work for me. In the same way Daisy establishes her attached focus with her eyes and body as her determination sets in, so have I done with romantic relationships. I can almost picture my posture being like Daisy's, my eyes set, vision narrowed, senses gone. All I see is what I have decided I want. And I have gone for it in the same wild and reckless ways Daisy has run toward dogs she does not know. Though neither of us has been bitten by doing so, unfortunate drama and pain have followed.

Lessons Learned

So what have I learned about being tenacious? It can be great and it can be trouble. I can get a lot accomplished, and I can leave a trail of problems in my wake. Daisy and Eddie certainly left some problems in their wake as they ran toward those poor, unsuspecting dogs and people. Again, no physical harm was done, but all of us felt the psychological effects for the rest of that day. Our dogs were confined to our car with only the basic food and occasional walks. The joy of our family outing was dampened, and we each quieted our self and did our own thing. We have no idea of what the impact was on the other family, but we assume they, too, experienced ripple effects in the form of assorted emotions throughout their day.

Learning about my tenacity has been more difficult than I want it to be. The problem is that I am, in some ways, attached to being tenacious. I could say it is part of my personality style, but so what? I know that it can go too far and needs to be moderated with mindfulness. So let's say that's the first lesson:

Tenacity can go too far and needs to be moderated with mindfulness.

Let's talk about these two parts separately.

Tenacity can go too far. As I have written above, being determined helps us to make things happen—good things, profitable things. But when it starts, as my husband says, "stepping on other people's toes," then it has gone too far. Interestingly enough, Daisy and Eddie were literally stepping on the toes of the other dogs and owners. When my focus is so narrowed on what I am determined about that I ignore or neglect other important people and things, including my healthier self, then I am carrying it too far, and I should not be surprised when negative consequences happen.

Tenacity needs to be moderated with mindfulness. If I am to change my tenacious behaviors so as to keep them from causing me problems, I need to continue to cultivate my awareness of my determination as it sets in and progresses. I cannot lose my self in my attachment to work, to someone else, to an idea, or to any number of other things. I need to be aware of the feelings building up inside me that drive me toward that goal I have set and mindfully be with them so I can make a balanced choice about whether to continue my pursuit in that moment or to take a break, step aside, pause, or just plain stop.

I can work toward the same purposes without an attack mode. I do not have to let go of what I am so determined about. I can work toward running my business well, writing another book, fixing up our old house, getting our finances in order. Daisy and Eddie could have met the other dogs if they had approached the situation calmly. It's the attacking posture that can cause trouble. Remember, the subtitle of this section says, "I know you want me to stop, but I don't want to." To reduce the attack factor, I must change this "I don't want to stop" part of me.

I need to adopt the value of stopping before it's too late. Notice the use of the word *value* here. That is what I have come to understand. I need to value stopping as much as I value keeping on. I need to see that knowing when to stop is an important part of getting to my goal, not an obstacle to it. My obsessive-compulsive style pushes the value of "productivity," and I don't like to be interrupted or stopped before I get to the point I have determined I need to get to. So let's keep the notion of stopping always in mind as we push on. And let's cultivate specific internal awareness of the cues that say, "You should stop now."

Stop now. The act of actually stopping is yet another challenge. I can tell my self all sorts of reasons and excuses for not stopping now, for finishing one more thing, for telling one more story. I need to continue to develop another voice within me that speaks, through self-talk, as loudly, clearly, and wisely and says,

"Really, stop now. You will be glad you did. You can continue later. Or not."

Because this stopping my self is such a challenge, I have several more lessons to reinforce the value of stopping when I am progressing from determined to controlling to rigid to compulsive:

Leave well enough alone. Many years ago I had gone to see a play with Grace and a friend of mine. The theater was full of people. There were no reserved seats, so we sat where we could. The seats we chose were farther back than I usually like, so I kept looking from my seat to see if I could find better seats for the three of us. Grace and my friend, however, were completely happy with where we were seated, and after a short time of dealing with me trying to locate something better for us, they said, "Nancy, leave well enough alone." I did. And I have held on deeply to this guideline that so clearly says to me that I don't need to do more. In fact, if I try to do more I may make things worse, not better. Perhaps things are "well enough" already.

Let go. All of this is really about letting go. Over and over I get to practice letting go. I let go of one more question, one more comment, one more suggestion, one more errand, one more stop at one more store. Truly this can all have compulsivity about it, and truly this letting go of these drives is greatly helped by the many aspects of my recovery including my mindfulness, my commitment to change, and my spirituality. When I am not letting go, I am acting out of my own willfulness and have disconnected from my higher power and the strength and wisdom that is there for me all the time. When I am not letting go, I am actually holding onto the wrong thing: I am holding onto what I want and not holding onto my spirituality, which can support me as I discern when, where, and how to stop my self in my pursuits that may involve things not even in my control.

"That'll do." Again I say what a lovely message this is. It conveys "Good job!" and "You can stop." How wonderful that the border collie learns this command. I am sure it makes its work with its shepherd sane and productive. I am sure that it also affords the border collie the reasonable opportunity to stop its work and to rest. I need to keep learning more about doing this and practice it.

Daisy, Eddie, and I all need more training in moderating our tenacity. These changes in our styles of determination and attachment are not necessarily easy to make. Perhaps these behaviors are central to our being; perhaps they are learned. Likely it is some of both. Either way, our health depends on our learning to moderate them, so we can live in civilized ways with our self and others. Training is necessary to teach all of us old dogs new tricks, and I assure you we all continue to get more training.

That'll do, Daisy.
That'll do, Eddie.
That'll do, Nancy.

delighted

•••••••••••••••••••••••••◄

*"I can be quite
pleased with
little things."*

Characteristic Described

I am adding "Delighted" to the list of qualities shared by the border collie and the codependent. I do not believe I have ever seen "delighted" on a list of codependent characteristics, but obviously I see a place for it.

Delighted means very pleased; delightful means very pleasing; a delight gives great pleasure. My experience with codependence is that many of us have good energy and spirit for life. We enjoy what we do. We are inspired and energetic. We are enthusiastic and see possibilities. Within us are ideas and intentions that have us out doing and creating with energy and meaning.

I put this quality on my original list of shared characteristics between Daisy and me as I first started working on this book in 2002. This similarity was easy to see as Daisy has a beautiful, happy face and always looks like she is smiling. She has a cute bounce to her step and likes to lick people with whom she is close. I identify with this type of good energy and spirit. I, too, am often feeling happy about my life. I am sure I can have a bounce to my step, and I can feel glad to see and be with others—though I don't lick them.

Mary Burch does not use the word *delighted* either as she describes the border collie, but she does describe this good energy and spirit. One of the general characteristics she lists is "lively,"[42] and she states that the border collie is "energetic, alert, and eager."[43]

I like those words: energetic and eager. I, too, can be energetic and eager. And though these are strengths, they, too, can go too far and become codependent behaviors. My eager self can become my overinvolved self. I can be so intent upon a project that I take it over completely and then become mad that others are not doing their part. My eager self can lead me to overdoing and/or overextending so that in that process I hurt or exhaust my self. My eager self can have me overfunctioning in others' lives. I can be so excited about what I want for them or think is best for them that my misplaced delight has me living their lives and not my own.

Yes, all of these are familiar pictures of codependent behaviors. What I am highlighting here is our delighted, delightful self, which is fueling these behaviors. There is absolutely nothing wrong with being excited about things. Mary Burch tells us several times how important excitement is to the border collie. The border collie needs activities that are "fun and exciting. For border collies, novelty is highly reinforcing."[44] When the border collie is herding, excitement is afoot! For us codependents, though, when our delighted, eager, and energized self has us out herding what is not ours to herd, we likely encounter problems.

What I like about this quality, "delighted," is that it not only addresses this good energy and eagerness we know, but it is also directly connected to pleasing. As you see above, being very pleased and being very pleasing are the ways *delighted* and its related words are defined. So in my delightfulness, I feel very pleased. In my delightfulness, I may also contribute to pleasing others, as such good spirit can be contagious.

And once again, all of this can get twisted into codependent behaviors.

If my delightfulness has me "quite pleased with little things," this can be okay and it can also be troubling. Not asking for too much or not asking for more than is reasonable helps to keep me and my life in balance. It is great when a simple walk or a fifty-cent item from a yard sale can delight me so. But if this tendency to be pleased by so little has me receiving very little from others or ever watching for crumbs of kindness from others, then my easy-to-please self may be getting hurt at several levels. I may simply be like a plant that needs watering, or I may be decaying at my very roots, believing I am not worthy of being considered and respected by others. Small pleasures may delight me, and sometimes I may need more. My health depends on my knowing when I need more and seeking reliable and loving sources for my watering.

If my delightfulness gets attached to wanting others to feel equally pleased, this, too, can be troubling. A simple way I have run into this problem is when I have called someone to share some exciting news with him or her, and he or she has responded in a way that does not match my level of pleasure. When this happens I am often disappointed that the person is not as delighted as I am, and I may be sorry that I even called to share the news. I feel tangled with that person and may even let my reaction to his or her reaction cause a disagreement or let it take away from the pleasure I was experiencing when I first called. This can happen also when I am presenting an idea that I think is very good to someone else or when I have a plan that may involve someone else. Though my delightedness is a great experience for me, I must not let it run me into situations where my expectations are that the other person will be as highly pleased as I am.

Some of these difficulties that can come from our delightedness involve *external focusing*. In its healthy form, delight comes from within. It is a natural energy, excitement, eagerness, and pleasure that fosters good work, good relationships, and a good self. But when our delight gets attached to wanting to delight others, then we have to be careful that our loss of self is not far away. We want to be able to maintain our internal inspirations and be careful not to shift into being dependent on people and things outside of our self for our inspiration. Codependents report they are bored or empty without problems of others to solve. They are described as getting their satisfaction and pleasure from satisfying and pleasing others. Through these behaviors, sources of delight become external, and the internal light of delight can become dimmed or go out. These behaviors are also about *interpersonal control,* which has us believing we can make things better for others and bring them the pleasure we know and want them to have.

There can be another layer of tangles when the delight we feel is dependent on other people experiencing the same or greater level of delight. It is almost as if they need to validate our delight to make our delight real rather than trusting and enjoying our own delight for what it is. Is it okay to feel this way? Is it okay to feel this good? How can I feel this good if you don't? This involves a variation on *emotional suppression* where we may be connected with our feelings but are not able to trust them without someone else giving us permission to do so. Or, in the reverse, with delight we also need to be mindful to notice if our delightedness is in fact obscuring additional feelings or even feelings contradictory to our delight. In our codependence, we can be so intent on the positive feelings of delight that we are unwilling to also acknowledge feelings that seem to us to hamper such pleasure.

Tales Told

Several months ago I took Daisy to see her veterinarian. It was time for her to have a checkup, and especially with her being sixteen years old, it is extra-important for me to keep up with her health needs. While she was doing her examination of Daisy, Dr. Keating asked me how this book was coming along. I reported my good progress and my delight with this work. With a strong understanding of what this book is about, Dr. Keating fell into a quick role-play with me of the border collie. She lowered her posture into the intense border collie stance and eye and said to me, "Throw me the ball! Throw me the ball! Throw me the ball!" Then she said, "We throw the border collie the ball, it runs and gets it and comes back and again says, 'Throw me the ball! Throw me the ball! Throw me the ball!'"

I spontaneously took the same border collie stance and eye to Dr. Keating and said, on behalf of the codependent, "Let me help! Let me help! Let me help!"

We both laughed and knew that we had just described the essence of this book. And in particular, we had just described this eager delight. The border collie is lively and delighted with work and engagement in fun activities. So is the codependent. What our role-play also highlighted, though, was the intensity of these feelings. Dr. Keating and I were practically face-to-face as we played this out with Daisy waiting somewhat impatiently between us, and it was clear that we both meant unyielding business, business that could have us pestering each other until we got our way.

Yes, Daisy is a delighted soul, as I have chosen to know her. I have a wonderful tale to tell you that shows her delight and the ways it can go too far. But first I want to tell you more about why I experience her as delightful. I have kept a list of things about Daisy and her life to write about in this book. Many of the things on that list have already been included, and yet when I was preparing for this chapter, it was notable to me how many of the items on the list remained, because so many of them are about the topic "Delighted."

A good place to start is to remind you that Grace says, "Daisy ran away from the circus to join a home!" And I often say, "Daisy, you make me smile." She is such a prancing little thing who trots along with ease and a happy smile. She easily gets excited and shows her delight by running in tight circles, jumping, or standing on her hind legs. She also shows her delight by some type of snuffling/sneezing sound she makes as her excitement mounts. Monty says she also does this when she is celebrating. How's that for a delightful word?

Daisy loves to roll on her back and rub it for a good while against our living room rug, on the remains of dead animals, or in manure. She is clearly in delight as she does this, and when she stops, she jumps up on her feet and gives her self a good, long shake, almost as if she is coming back into reality after the ecstasy of her experience.

Daisy is truly "quite pleased with little things." Occasionally we will give her small scraps, and you would think we were giving her pounds of meat. Somewhere along the line we started letting Daisy and Eddie chew up the cardboard tube from an empty roll of toilet paper. Daisy will come into the bathroom and stare at the toilet paper roll, obviously hoping that soon the empty tube will be hers to enjoy.

And then there are those simple, endearing qualities and behaviors about Daisy that I love:

The tags on Daisy's collar have a little jingle to them as she moves. I can hear her coming, and I am pleased.

She has a deliberate and quiet way of coming up the stairs to join me.

At least once a day she goes into an excited fit of running up against the side of our sofas, back and forth, rubbing her self as she goes, snuffling, sneezing, and then shaking her self well when she is done.

When lying under our kitchen table, Daisy rests her chin on the cross-braces of the chairs pushed under the table, and when she is standing, she rests her chin on a footstool or sofa cushion. She appears both restful and attentive. We always smile at this, not really knowing why she does it but being delighted by her posture and her presence in our life.

Daisy does bring us pleasure, and she truly has pleasure and delight within her. A walk down to the river always reveals this. With her eager prancing and running toward our delta, it is clear how happy she feels. But even this wonderful delight in going to the river can go too far as my tale, "Up the River: A Tale on Us Both," will show.

In 2010, Jim, Grace's English boyfriend, was staying with us for several weeks in May and early June before he left to go up to the Adirondack Mountains in New York state, where he and Grace both work at a summer camp for the arts. We were so glad to have him with us, and I really wanted to show him a nice time. As you know, we live on the river, so I thought that some activities on the water would be a great idea.

Prior to Jim's visit, I had purchased an inflatable kayak as a gift for Monty. Honestly, I suppose it was a gift for me, since I was the one so excited about it, but I had given it to Monty for his birthday. I decided that Jim might like to try the kayak. The river is slow enough in front of our place that we are able to paddle our canoe or tubes upstream for a good way and then float back to home. I thought Jim might like to do this, and he said he would.

So we pulled the kayak out of the attic and inflated it in our living room with our hand pump. I remember being all happy and energetic about this outing for us all. The border collie in me was already rallied and ready to herd everyone to the river and have them enjoy themselves as much I was. The dogs were picking up on this energy as well, and as we walked out of the front door with the kayak, towels, chairs, and sunglasses, they bolted down to the river.

Once we were all there, Jim got into the kayak and started to get the feel of it. Since it is a lightweight boat, there is an art to paddling it in a way to keep it going straight. We explained the simple terrain to him of paddling upriver, giving him a description of a class-one rapid he would paddle through that would then enable him to travel farther until he reached a class-two rapid, at which point we usually turn around and float home. Jim said, "Fine," and he was off.

And without our permission, Daisy was off on the adventure as well! As we had prepared Jim, she was eagerly watching us all from the riverbank. Over the years, Daisy has ridden in our canoe with us and been allowed to get out of the canoe at times and run along the bank. She loves to do this. And as she watched our activities getting Jim ready to go, she assessed that this was a trip for her, too.

There are a couple of things to note as I tell this story. First, at the time of this adventure, Daisy was in her fifteenth year of life. So although she had good energy and strength, she was an old dog. And second, Jim was a strong young man who was able to move that kayak swiftly upstream.

So off they went. We tried to call Daisy back, but she ignored us. Jim was paddling close enough to the bank that he could hear us and see her for a while and shout back that she was with him. The bank has full-grown trees and brush all along it, making it not possible to always see Daisy unless she runs down to the river's edge. So although Jim was doing his best to watch for her, he really could not supervise her.

I was standing on our delta watching all of this, watching my delight and excitement morph into concern and anxiety. I did not like Daisy off and running madly up the river while Jim, whom she hardly knew was supposed to be having a great time floating on the river. We were all shouting to Jim and gesturing in ways that conveyed no meaning. And then he was out of sight around the bend.

I was starting to be beside my self with concern. Daisy was out of control. Her delight had run away with her, and she had run away from us. Reason seemed to have disappeared, as did her training. In addition to all of this disorder, the railroad track runs along this riverbank and trains regularly use it, so as I worried about where Daisy was, the train track was another one of my concerns.

Not long after he went around the bend, we saw Jim coming back down the river. He was moving along more swiftly now, because he was going with the flow of the current. We started our shouting and unclear gesturing again, trying to determine if Daisy was with him. He couldn't hear us or understand us. My upset was mounting, as I did not know what was going on with Daisy at all. Finally Jim was within earshot, and he let us know that he had no idea where Daisy was. He had not seen her for a while, nor did he hear her running through the brush on the bank.

That did it! My action was required! Monty said he was going to go up to our property and get the canoe. I watched Jim coming back to our delta with my border collie eye, intent on only him and that kayak he was in that I now wanted. Jim, who has a calm and centered demeanor, paddled up to the shore where Grace and I stood, and reported that he last saw Daisy somewhere around the bend of the river, running along the bank.

With focused purpose, I took the kayak paddle from Jim, hopped in the kayak, and took off upstream as I never had before. I was paddling like I was a strong, twenty-three-year-old male. I was staying as close to the bank as I could, knowing this is where the current is weaker and where Daisy might be. And I started yelling for her to come.

I yelled and yelled: "Daisy, Come!" "Daisy, Come!" "Daisy,

Come!" I am sure I must have looked like a madwoman in that silly little inflatable kayak, trying to reach Olympic speeds upriver, shouting all the way.

I got around the bend and through the class-one rapid. No sign of Daisy. On the rock beach on the other side of the river were some of our neighbors, also out to enjoy the river. One of them was sitting in a lawn chair in the water, all calm and peaceful. She shouted over to me, asking what was going on. I explained that I was missing Daisy and asked if she had seen her. She said yes, that Daisy had been on my side of the river heading up to the class-two rapid a while ago. Good news and not good news. Daisy had been sighted, but that sighting was old.

My neighbor volunteered to get her car and drive on the roads near this stretch of the river. I declined her offer, trying not to make a complete emergency out of this situation. But it was an emergency for me. This I knew. Yet I also had kept enough awareness of my self to know that I was likely reacting too strongly to the situation at this point. Yes, Daisy is old and can't see or hear very well. Yes, Daisy is not allowed to run free like this. She is always under our supervision. But I did not have to be so catastrophic. In fact, my dramatic shift from delight to catastrophe was not helpful at all. This awareness of my self allowed me to respond to my neighbor's offer in a civilized way, but it did not stop the internal process of anxiety and disaster from filling me as much as my delight had filled me in our living room as we prepared to come play on the river.

I kept paddling frantically and calling for her with earnest love. I did not see or hear her. The bank seemed hauntingly quiet and empty. I could not believe it. I could not believe Daisy was gone. I could not believe that she had become so consumed by her pleasures that she had run away with them.

Then I wondered if I'd heard someone call my name. I quieted my insane paddling that was throwing water right and left, right and left. I quieted my shouting of "Daisy! Daisy!" I looked to each side of the river and saw no one. My neighbors, now behind me, had resumed their calm appreciation of the day and the river. I saw no one coming from upriver toward me.

"Nancy! Nancy! Nancy!"

"Momma! Momma! Momma!"

I looked behind me, and there in the distance, coming upriver toward me, was our canoe with Monty, Grace, Jim, Eddie, AND Daisy all aboard. The dogs were in the front of the canoe, all happy with eager panting and tails wagging. Daisy looked as pleased as she could be, and was especially pleased that she could see me and know that we would soon be together.

Or was it me who was pleased now that I could see her and know that we would soon be together? I believe it was both. I was frantically relieved. I had thought I would never see Daisy again. I had thought she was gone for good. She was so out of my control, and then I became nearly out of my control. What a ridiculous pair we can be.

When we all came together in the river, Monty reported to me that as he, Grace, Jim, and Eddie had made their way up the river behind me, Daisy simply showed up somewhere along the riverbank and asked for them to come pick her up. She had had enough of, as Monty calls it, her insane adventure and was able and ready to rejoin her family. Fortunately, she could. Fortunately, she had not run into trouble with her old legs, her poor hearing, or the railroad tracks.

I, too, had had enough of my insane adventure, and, fortunately for me, I had Daisy back.

Lessons Learned

If this is not a story about delight going too far, I don't know what is. Old Daisy Dog ran a couple of miles upriver and back, completely disconnecting from her family and her training. She threw caution to the river. And I ran after her with the same intensity and near-disconnect from self and reason. It is as if the river is a continuum, and we can easily see Daisy and me traveling on up that continuum from delighted at our house and delta to insanity somewhere between the class-one and class-two rapids. Except that Daisy and I did not only lose our selves in this adventure, but also, it is important to note, both of us found our way back to our selves, and our being both lost and found enables me to offer these lessons:

Life can be delightful. I know this from my personal experience. I have always been blessed with being able to feel highly pleased about things, big and small. I can remember as a little girl being told by my parents that we would be doing something, such as running to the store or raking leaves, and I would get excited about whatever it was. I could imagine the possibilities even in raking leaves and making forts out of the piles. Life has endless treats for us all of the time. Yes, we know it also has surprises that disrupt and disturb us, but I believe it is important to acknowledge that we can be delighted at any moment by any little thing, and I want to be open to those moments and experience them. These are not moments I have to create. These are moments that are there for my noticing and pleasure as an extension of my noticing.

I enjoy feeling delighted. I know and trust this feeling. It is okay for me to feel delighted. It is important for me to feel delighted. Sometimes our life experiences have taught us to calm down and not be so excited. Sometimes our anxiety wants to step in and say, "Now wait a minute. You can't feel this good. There are things to be worried about or to feel bad about." It wants to overshadow the wonderfulness of delight. I want to remind my self that it is completely okay for me to feel these positive feelings, and I want to use self-talk and mindfulness to support my experience of delight when these other messages to self challenge my pleasure.

Good things can come from my delight. When I am feeling this pleasure and excitement, it can naturally create more pleasure and excitement. We all know that we can walk into a room and feel tension when there has been an argument or disagreement among the people already there in the room. The same can be true with good feelings. We know when we have come into a space where there is laughter and lightness and kindness. The delight in that space feels good and refreshing and lightens us. My delight inspires me, giving me ideas I've never had before and energy to do what I have in mind. My delight allows me to see others more fully and lovingly, and my acceptance of my self and others is strengthened.

I can't make others experience the same delight that I am experiencing. Yes, my good feelings have the potential to spill into a space and change or improve the feelings of other people there, but I had best not have that as my agenda. My delight is *my* delight. When I try to get others to feel the same way, I am setting my self up for tangles, as I have no control over how they feel. I feel my feelings and they feel theirs. When I am trying to make someone else as excited as I am about something and I am not succeeding at doing so, there's a good chance that now I am not so excited anymore either. What a loss for me.

I can feel delight even when others don't feel it. Now I don't want to be obnoxious about my delight in the face of someone else not experiencing it as I am, but I don't want to negate my good feelings just because the other person does not have the same reaction as I am having. I want to remember that I have my own feelings, that it is important for me to be in touch with my own feelings, and that it is okay for me to express my own feelings. Delight happens to be one of those feelings. I don't want to be dependent on the other person having the same level of delight as mine in order for me to trust that my feelings of delight are real and valid. I want my trust of my feelings to come from within me.

I can lose my self in intense delight. In the same way that I do not want to lose my self in bad experiences and feelings, letting them affect my total sense of self, I do not want to lose my self in good feelings, either. When I lose my self in this way, I am disconnecting from other important information about my self and others and the situations at hand. This is actually like being intoxicated with my delight—drunk, quite frankly—and we know the unmanageability that drunkenness brings. We know the regrets that drunkenness brings as well. I don't want to be drunk with delight. It does not serve me well. I do not serve my self well in being so intoxicated.

I don't want my delight to obscure my reason. My delight can interfere with my thinking. It can either have me not thinking clearly or it can have me not thinking at all. My great pleasure can bias my thinking, causing me to make decisions I might not make otherwise. It might have me believing things that are not true, or it may invite me to not think about what is true right now. Whatever form it takes, I have learned that while I experience my delight, it is important that I also stay connected with my thinking brain and maintain a level of willingness to listen to it. I may feel like my thoughts are interfering with my great feelings. I do not want to let that interference happen unnecessarily, and at the same time, I do not want to let my extreme delight damage my good judgment.

I don't want my delight to obscure my other feelings. In the same way that my delight can interfere with my thinking, it can also interfere with my ability to connect with other feelings I may be simultaneously having. Some of those feelings may even be in direct conflict with the excitement and pleasure that are dominant then. Again, it can be tricky and challenging to sort out whether these other feelings are trying unnecessarily to keep me from feeling delight or are important warning signs for me that I have drunk enough delight for now. I want to be able to acknowledge and feel those other feelings and determine where they are coming from and what to do to respond as authentically to them as I am responding to my delight.

I don't want my delight to have me accepting too little. And I certainly don't want my delight to have me accepting the unacceptable. Once again I am teasing apart some important but sometimes subtle differences between what I am willing to accept for my self and what I am not. I want to be careful to not have expectations of others that trip me up and disappoint me. At the same time, I do not want to be treated in neglectful and/or abusive ways that eat away at my sense of self. I do not want my delight in small, occasional experiences to be enough to hold me in a relationship that is not good for my self. I do not want my ability to see delightful possibilities in another person or in my relationships with others to keep me from also seeing the realities of people and situations.

My eagerness and excitement are welcome and are best accompanied by my awareness of my full self and situation. As I experience my eagerness and excitement, I want to be paying attention to all four areas of my self: feeling, thinking, physical, and spiritual. I want to be able to acknowledge the other feelings that may be accompanying my delight. I want to be able to think clearly and honestly. I want to notice what my body is telling me, too. Is it upset? Is it saying, "Calm down"? Is it saying, "Get out of here"? Is it relaxed? And, as always, I want to connect with my spirit. My delight can rob me of this connection if I am not mindful. It can take over and mislead me into believing that my delight is my spiritual experience, when in fact my delight has become my drug of choice. Through mindful pauses, intentional contact with my higher power, and true willingness and honesty with my self, I can fully enjoy my delight without losing my self in it. Somewhere along her runaway experience upriver, Daisy sobered up from her delight, turned around, and started coming home. She came to the bank of the river and caught her canoe ride back to the solid ground of her home. That's what I want to be able to do as well, so that I am not paddling upriver like a madwoman, shouting in desperation to empty riverbanks.

big-hearted

....

*"I love you dearly
and will follow you
anywhere."*

Characteristic Described

"Big-hearted" appeared on the original list of characteristics Daisy and I share that I wrote on April 6, 2002, on a notepad in the Cavalier Hotel in Virginia Beach, Virginia. Grace, Monty, and I were in this oceanfront hotel as Monty was doing service work for his twelve-step fellowship, which was meeting there. Daisy was with us, too. I remember sitting at the window of our room a number of floors up overlooking the ocean and writing this list, already entitled "My Life as a Border Collie." The list came easily and logically and meaningfully. "Big-hearted" was the eighth item, and beside it I wrote "spirit."

For me this word *spirit* and its relationship to Daisy means several things. I see Daisy as having a good spirit, as having love and kindness and good energy. When she comes into a room, she brightens it. When she wants to go do something, she eagerly prances around with her request, making us smile. And she certainly does follow me around with devotion. That was another reason I readily added "big-hearted" to the list; as Daisy regularly conveys, "I love you dearly and will follow you anywhere."

"Big-hearted" does not usually appear on lists describing codependents, but I believe it is an important attribute that underlies many of our other codependent behaviors. In its pure form, I believe being big-hearted is truly an asset. The dictionary actually has a listing for *big-hearted*. It is defined as being "generous; charitable." In further investigations of these common words, I found that *generous* is defined as "liberal in giving," and *charitable* as "full of love and goodwill for others."* I like these definitions very much. They are indeed what I have in mind when I put "big-hearted" on this list.

I have my own ways of expressing this big-heartedness as well. I think of being big-hearted as being generously and positively spirited. I think of it as being loyal, kind, thoughtful, and giving. I believe that this giving that comes from being big-hearted is offered genuinely and freely. This is big-hearted in its pure form: What we are offering from the goodness of our hearts is not looking for something to come back to us as a result our giving. We are offering something because we want to offer it, and our offering is not attached to any expectations from or of others. It is a free, heartfelt gift.

Mary Burch describes this big-heartedness in the border collie in several ways. "Loyal" appears on a list of seven characteristics presented in a side box as a primary description of this breed.[45] In another list of characteristics describing the temperament of the border collie, she states that this dog is "affectionate toward friends" and "thrives on human companionship."[46]

In speaking of their willingness to please, Mary Burch further explains, "When they are paired with an owner who understands the breed and what it takes to work with a dog that is so mentally and physically alert, the relationship can be beautiful."[47] I am particularly

---

*By permission. From *Merriam-Webster's Collegiate® Dictionary*, 11th Edition ©2012 by Merriam-Webster, Incorporated (www.Merriam-Webster.com).

struck by the description of the relationship as "beautiful." For me, that's what much of my recovery from codependency is about. I want to have a beautiful relationship with my self and with others. I believe that is my big-heartedness that is speaking in wanting this goodness. So how, with such a wish for love and goodwill, can I go wrong? Looking at several of the defining features of codependency can help us to better understand the tangles that can come from being big-hearted.

First let's look at *external focusing* in the work of Dear, Roberts, and Lange[48] and Dear and Roberts.[49] Remember, this behavior involves focusing on the behaviors, opinions, and expectations of other people and trying to adjust our self to fit with others. In its more extreme form, this behavior involves being so focused on the other person that we neglect our other relationships and responsibilities and our very self. Such focusing can have us feeling empty and unworthy if we are not so intimately involved with someone else. These do not sound like beautiful relationships to me. Being big-hearted can lead us in this direction of unhealthiness in a couple of ways. If our love and kindness and generosity are tied to an excessive extent to the wanting to obtain approval and acceptance from others that can be involved in *external focusing,* then we may be creating problems for our self. If our loyalty and good spirit are not genuinely and freely offered to this external object of our attention, then we are setting our self up for troubled feelings and conflicts in our relationships. We can have our external focus, but as we do this and offer our gifts of love and kindness and giving, we had best note if somewhere in there we are also seeking something back from the other person in return for our offerings.

Self-sacrificing is also a danger for us in our big-heartedness. *Self-sacrificing* in its more extreme form has us neglecting our needs in order to meet the needs of others. We place the needs of others ahead of our own. We tell our self that what we feel and need is not important as long as everybody else has everything they need. Being big-hearted can feed this self-sacrificing if we are not mindful. We can lose our self in our generosity and giving. We can get so excited and be so pleased by all of the good feelings coming from our good works that we lose our connection with our self. In "Delighted" I spoke about becoming intoxicated with our delight; I believe we can become intoxicated by the feelings and actions that come from our being big-hearted as well. In this process, we lose touch with other parts of our self and will likely, at some point, have a hangover from all of our giving and the consequences that can come from our overextension of our time, money, emotions, and resources.

Woven into this picture of how "big-hearted" can go wrong is *interpersonal control*: the belief that we can fix and control others. Well, already I see the problematic setup: Big-hearted can be about wanting to fix others. It can be about wanting to make things better for others. It is often about this type of giving of help. I am certainly not proposing that we stop such acts of kindness. I am, however, saying that our behaviors move from being generous and charitable to being codependent when our giving is deeply attached to making sure that we fix things for others or make things better for them. These giving behaviors on our part become codependent when we believe we know what is best for others and try to impose that on them. We are acting codependently when we give something someone else has said he or she does not want. We are acting codependently when our sense of self is dependent on our success at making things better for someone else. We are acting codependently when our being big-hearted has intentions of fixing and controlling rather than freely giving.

And I am acting codependently when I go so far as to be willing to risk life and limb unnecessarily in order to show and share my big-heartedness. Such a near-complete loss of self can be dangerous, as my tales about Daisy and I will show. We both "love you dearly and will follow you anywhere," and we both have been known to carry this too far.

Tales Told

As I have established, Daisy does follow me everywhere. I spoke of this in the "Devoted" chapter and return to this behavior here. Daisy's attention to me and her movement with me from room to room in our house did inspire my ideas for this book, noting her attachment to me shown in these ways. I choose to see this attachment as coming from her big-hearted love for me. And I know I feel this big-hearted love for her.

When I come upstairs to write in the mornings, Daisy comes upstairs, too, and lies on the floor at my feet.

When I return downstairs, usually to the kitchen, Daisy comes, too, and hangs out with me as I work.

When we go out on walks, Daisy does a good job of paying attention to where I am and checking back in with me periodically.

When we go sit on the sofa to watch a movie, Daisy comes, too, and lies at my feet.

When I go upstairs to go to bed, Daisy realizes this and comes along with me, lying down on her foam mattress beside my side of the bed.

"Daisy, I keep you busy," I am inclined to say to her as we move from one activity of the day to another. There is no doubt that Daisy is my loyal companion, sharing her love and laughter with me as we go through the day together. She is always nearby.

I adore this good-spirited relationship with Daisy. As I have told you before, I am Daisy's main person. So I am the one who receives most of this attentive love. I wish others could experience her more in these ways, but this is, in part, about her breed, and we have come to accept this. In an interesting way, this can be true of codependence as well, with our entire focus being on one person so that others fade from our view and from our hearts. So in this way, Daisy's big-heartedness is not perfect and is sometimes a problem in that she may ignore others if I am around or refuse to do what someone else is asking of her.

Recently I also started to see how Daisy's being big-hearted can cause problems with her physical health. I call this brief tale "Risking Life and Limb."

I have told you how eagerly Daisy greets me when I come home from work at night. Monty, Daisy, and Eddie come out the front door as soon as I have backed the car into the driveway and turned it off. Both dogs come flying off the front porch, running toward me with great delight. And I am delighted. It is a fine greeting and reunion that has never gone so far as to cause problems, as I explained in the chapter on "Hardworking."

Several weeks ago, however, Daisy was full of extra enthusiasm as we all greeted one another. She went into her agility run around my car, making a couple of laps with me smiling and cheering her on. Seeing her happy energy and amazing physical talents, even at her age, makes me so happy, too.

Then Daisy ran over to what we call "the structure," not too far away from my car. This structure used to be a tipple, a place where railroad cars could back in and be loaded with ore from the valley on the other side of our river. What remains of this structure are large concrete walls that rise up from a concrete floor elevated about four feet off the ground. Over the past year, I have been developing this unusual space by creating a garden-bed-and-shed there with patio spaces for planting and sitting. Daisy can easily get up and down from the structure by using garden paths from either end, which run up to the structure's four-foot level, and she has been enjoying getting up there more and more as I have been making it a nice place to be.

So Daisy ran over to the structure, easily accessing it through one of the end paths. I walked over to the structure to speak to this energized dog. When I stand on the ground by the structure, I am able to see Daisy eye to eye. Daisy was prancing back and forth along the edge of the structure. She came over to me, we kissed, and she trotted around to the shed. I thought she was headed toward the other end of the structure, where she usually gets off by going down the leafy bank. I was about to walk back to my car to get my stuff out when Daisy ran back to where I was standing beside the structure and leaped off the structure to the ground!

I was standing right beside her as she made this six-foot leap through space. I could not do anything. I could not believe it was happening. I had never seen or known Daisy to do this Evel Knievel stuff off of our structure. I had certainly seen her leap off lower and softer surfaces, such as porches, steps, and the banks along our paths. But I had not seen her attempt such a gigantic, death-defying airborne stunt. In that moment of watching her fly through space, I feared for her life. I could not imagine how her sixteen-year-old body, which is eighty-seven years old in human years, could possibly not be harmed by this leap of love. I had tried so hard to take good care of her, and now, in this moment of big-heartedness gone wild, Daisy had risked life and limb.

I watched Daisy land on the uneven ground several feet away from me. She made a small yelp as she hit and ran on toward the front door of our house, ready for me to follow and to give her a treat for being a good dog. I tried to check her out for any injury from the impact, nervously telling Monty what had just happened while he was in the house, and explaining the importance of our watching her for a while to make sure we didn't see any residual problems from her acrobatics.

We have not seen any problems. Daisy hasn't even shown a

limp from her leap. For this I am beyond glad. But what a disturbing moment that truly was for me as I stood right beside my dear companion and watched helplessly as she let her love for having me home lead her to taking such a dangerous leap, seemingly beyond what her body could have tolerated.

*   *   *   *   *

Dangerous leaps of love. That's what I'm talking about—love expressed in ways that risk harm to self and/or to others. Certainly there are times when our love for someone else demands extreme measures on our part to help or to save him or her. But most of the time, our big-heartedness does not require us to make decisions that put us or others at risk of harm.

My next tale does not reflect these extremes of risk, but it does show questionable judgment on my part as I showed Grace "I love you dearly and will follow you anywhere." I'll call this tale "The Big Brass Bed."

Grace left home for college in the fall of 2006. It was not a happy time for any of us. Though our household had certainly had its various levels of insanity as Grace grew up, the three of us loved one another and spent much time together around the house and while traveling. As we were all leaving to take her to college her freshman year, Grace said, "I feel like I am going to my funeral." That's how powerful our separating was for each of us. We all knew the importance of this necessary change and did nothing to delay or avoid it, but it was not easy for us. We knew we could not let our love for Grace have us following her to college. We had to let her go to this next level of self-development, and we had to grow into our own next level of separation and individuation as well.

Grace lived in a residence hall her freshman year. At the end of that year, Grace found a small, sweet apartment for her self to live in during her sophomore year. It was a single apartment in the heart of the campus. Monty and I were fine with this plan, but I noticed that I started to make it *my* plan, even though Grace was fully and competently in charge of finding, securing, and furnishing this place of her own. I went to graduate school at this same university and had lived in this same charming part of the city. I have a love for the old townhouses there and for fixing them up. I am also a codependent.

Because of my recovery, however, I was able to not take over Grace's plans. I knew the importance of empowering her. I have my own home to fix up. She now had hers. I was able to not take over . . . for the most part.

In the August before Grace was to return to college for her sophomore year and to her new apartment, I was driving to my office in town and went by a house on a nice street in Lexington where the owner had put a queen-size brass bed with a box spring and mattress to the curb for the taking. I couldn't believe it. We had not yet decided what to do about a bed for Grace in her apartment, though I was letting that go, too, for her to figure out.

The bed and all of its fixings were resting against a big tree. I could not stop to check it out, because I had no extra time before my first appointment of the day, but I knew I wanted that bed! I wanted that bed like crazy! It was charming, inviting, good quality, and just what I would want for Grace. I knew I would feel really good setting her up in her apartment with such a fine place to rest. She would be just like a princess!

So in between my appointments that morning, I made a couple of calls to secure my getting that bed. Ours is a small community, so, since I knew other people who lived on the street, I was able to call around, find out whose bed it was, and call them. I also called Grace, who was receptive to the idea but not nearly as overcome with it as I was. That did not stop me.

Later that day, Grace joined me briefly for us to go see the bed close up. We were very pleased, and the owner was glad for it to have a great home. The owner's complaint about it was that it had some looseness to the frame. Grace and I were able to move the bed, box spring, and mattress to the big Victorian front porch of the house next door, which just happened to be the home of her ex-boyfriend in high school. We have remained good friends with that family, and we knew they would not mind coming home and finding their neighbor's bed on their front porch with no more explanation than that. Grace got a screwdriver out of their garage and immediately fixed the problem that had caused this change of ownership.

This tale so far has shown glimpses of my efforts to let Grace grow up and to leave things for her to take care of that are hers to do. I could not follow her to college, but I wanted to be a part of her life there in whatever ways I could. I do not think there is anything wrong with this. I think this parental involvement is very natural. I do think we have to be mindful, though, that transitions are happening as our children grow and go, and I need to make sure I am not overinserting my self. If Grace had said no to the bed, I needed to be ready to accept her no.

But she did not say no. She said yes, and the rest of this tale is about the antics of Grace and me getting that queen-size bed from the Valley of Virginia to Richmond. In the next part of this tale, though I probably did not risk life and limb, I certainly did make questionable decisions. I do love Grace dearly, and my heart really does want to follow her anywhere. But since I can't follow her everywhere, I can get caught up in trying to make her life as happy and comfortable as I want it to be for her, wherever she is. When it comes to Grace, I am very big-hearted. Ah, the lengths we will go to for those we love.

Grace and I decided that, considering our resources, the only way for us to get the brass head- and footboards, railings, box spring, and mattress to Richmond was to borrow a minivan from our good friends. They are very generous with sharing their vehicles, and we knew this minivan would also provide us with additional space for the many other household possessions Grace would be taking.

Some days after acquiring the bed, Monty, Grace, and I came to get it off our friends' front porch. We arrived with the minivan, big sheets of plastic, ropes, bungee cords, and duct tape. We worked for a long time in their driveway, trying to figure out the best way to carry all of this. We had hoped that the head- and footboards would fit inside the van, but they did not. It became clear that we needed to stack all of these parts of the bed on top of the van and secure them.

Monty had to work that night, so only Grace and I were traveling with this load. It was a sunny day. Our trip was around 150 miles and involved traveling mostly on interstate highways. It also involved going over the Blue Ridge Mountains, where there can be more wind, and on beltways around Richmond where there can be crazy, heavy traffic. I am a good, seasoned driver, having shared long-distance driving with Monty on three round-trips across the USA. But I am not a cargo carrier and have little to no experience with driving with a tall load on the top of my vehicle. My anxiety started to mount as the load on our roof mounted.

We did not find it easy to place, wrap, and secure all of these parts of the bed on the top of the minivan. I remember us having tense, conflicted moments about how to do it. I also remember having no good ideas my self about the best way to attach all of this. I knew we were piecing our plan together in ways that did not make me confident about our safety and the bed's security.

Nevertheless, we did the best we could, Grace and I got in the van, and we drove out of the driveway. Slowly traveling down this residential street, we were fine at ten or fifteen miles per hour, but as soon as we went over those speeds, the plastic, which was protection in case of rain, started rattling and the front edges of the load, which I could see above the windshield, started bouncing. We had not even gone one mile, and we knew we were in for a long trip. We laughed at the notion that we would drive all the way to Richmond at ten miles per hour. It seemed like a real possibility, though.

We made our way out to the bypass around Lexington, having gone two miles at this point. The speed limit on the bypass is fifty-five miles per hour. We could not even attempt that speed that without major disruption to our load, so we pulled over to the side of the road to assess our situation. We knew we had set sail on our trip; our load was acting like it was setting sail as well. Funny now, not funny then, though we did keep our sense of humor throughout.

Grace and I made a few adjustments to tighten the ropes holding the bed. The plastic was what had gone wild already. Every little place air could find, it had, and it had blown the plastic loose. We tried to contain it by pushing it under the ropes. We got back in the van and were able to drive one more mile when we were once again experiencing turbulence from the plastic flying around. Now, remember what an anxious person I have told you I can be. This type of situation is very challenging for my anxiety. I kept imagining all of the pieces of this wonderful bed flying backward off our roof and onto the road, landing right in front of the poor drivers behind us. But my love for Grace and my desire to get this bed to her apartment in Richmond were overriding my anxiety. These two powerful feelings were competing with each other and creating a real mental health challenge for me.

With one more mile traveled, Grace and I stopped again to assess and fix our load. We were fussing about our situation, dealing with the August sun bearing down on us, and trying to figure out what to do. We decided we needed to use more duct tape. Of course, life can always use more duct tape to make things better. And so we did. We used the rest of our roll to tape this crazy plastic so that it wouldn't billow out, rattle, and tear the entire load off the top of the van. We thought we were good and drove on. We went one more mile. The problems returned. We were right near a hardware store and decided to go in and buy more duct tape.

As we came out of the store with our duct tape, we realized that there was no need for all of this plastic anyway. It was a hot August day, with plenty of sun and no rain in the forecast. So, with great pleasure, we started taking the plastic off the box spring and mattress without untying anything. Fortunately for us we were traveling with other furniture in the van, so we got out a chair and a stool to use as our ladders. Removing the plastic was not particularly easy, as there were many ropes and bungee cords in use, and some of them ran through the windows, making it impossible to open some of our doors. In fact, we could not get all of the plastic off, but we got most of it, tearing it away happily. I am sure we were quite a picture in the parking lot with our stool, chair, and flying plastic. No one offered to help us through all of this. That's okay. I don't know how they could have helped us anyway. We really did not know what we were doing.

With the plastic mostly gone, we once again set sail, but without our sail. As we gained speed on our local road, which leads to the interstate, we could tell that the load was quieter and steadier. But I had lost my confidence through all of this. I was not convinced that everything would stay in place, and the remaining plastic still rattled and came loose at times. So I decided not to take the interstate highway, but rather to use our local roads for a while. I was determined to get the bed to Richmond. I was not turning back. Even though my anxiety, and some reality, had me believing that I was perhaps risking life and limb for this mission of love, I was not to be stopped.

We did get to Richmond safely many hours later. I carefully drove along at slower speeds, watching the activity on my roof as best as I could and periodically stopping to tighten the ropes. I would say that we hobbled to Richmond. We didn't stop for gas. We didn't stop for anything other than rope tightening. I was on this meager roll and wanted to keep going. I got on the interstate when it was time to go over the Blue Ridge Mountains, and I held my breath as we made it over the top with the winds blowing. As we got into the metropolitan area, I stayed in the right lane, paying hypervigilance to my load, not wanting to shift lanes or speeds abruptly or to go too fast.

As we exited the interstate, close to Grace's apartment, I remember feeling deep relief. I kept our silly, slow, cautious pace until we parked right in the front of her apartment building where we were greeted by Amy, Grace's best friend, who was there to help us move the bed into a tiny elevator and up five floors to Grace's place.

Would I do this again? Yes. Do I know what I could have done to make this trip less exciting and safer? No. Is that a problem? Yes. Though we all arrived safely and think this is now a funny tale to tell, I believe it also speaks to my insanity when I am letting my heart be in full control. I believe it shows me how being big-hearted can put me and others in danger, and it also shows the close interplay of being big-hearted with being devoted, hardworking, serving, pleasing, and tenacious. It probably shows the interplay of all of the behaviors I have written about in this book.

Whether it is an Evel Knievel stunt that has Daisy airborne or my willingness to be a highway safety threat, in these situations Daisy and I have let being big-hearted go too far. Our hearts have run away with us and all is not well.

I cannot afford to let my love for you have me following you just anywhere and doing just anything. This is an important lesson I have learned as a result of these stunts Daisy and I have pulled, and there are more lessons as well.

Lessons Learned

As I have been writing this chapter, I have realized that in some ways this book is now coming full circle. I started these Tales and Lessons with a chapter on "Smart." One of the things I highlighted there was the importance of not losing our self in our smartness, not letting our thinking self obscure other important parts of our self that also need to be heard and respected. In this chapter on "Big-hearted," an important message is for us to not lose our self in our feelings, either. Over and over, we are learning the importance of listening to our self in balanced ways that consider the thinking, feeling, physical, and spiritual parts of our self. Strength in any one of these areas can become a weakness if it dominates the ways we treat our selves and others. To this end, I have learned:

Being big-hearted is a gift. It is truly wonderful to be able to experience love, kindness, and generosity. These emotions make me feel very alive and connected to my life and the world around me. My big-heartedness inspires me to create and to give, to feel excitement and happiness. It takes me down paths on which I meet people I may not have met otherwise, or has me doing things I've never done before: good things, thoughtful things, meaningful things. What a gift to be able to live with such loving emotional experiences.

Giving genuinely and freely is rich. As I live with my big-heartedness, loving and giving to others is best done without any expectation of something coming back to me for my offerings. To this end, it is important that as I give, I need to check with my self to make sure I do, indeed, want to do or give whatever it is I have in mind and to note if I have any hopes attached to the outcome of my giving. If I don't genuinely want to give or do, then perhaps I should not. My giving is best done without imposing expectations on others. Setting up giving with "If I do ____, then I'll get ____" is not being big-hearted. It is a contractual relationship needing to be mutually established. Giving genuinely and freely comes from my heart, and its richness comes from the love and freedom I experience as I give and let go.

I do not want to be intoxicated by my love. I want to fully experience my feelings of love, kindness, and generosity, and at the same time, I do not want to be blinded by them. I do not want to lose my self in emotional states that come from being big-hearted. I do not want to let these emotions run away with me. I want to both fully experience them and have a "sobriety" within me at the same time. I want to feel them and yet not let them rush to my head, pushing out reason and spirit. Intoxication lasts only a while. It may feel good as it is happening, but many of us know that later we regret our drunkenness and its consequences. Such can be the case with the power of strong emotional states as well. I can overindulge in my big-heartedness and lose track of a lot of other important things, including and especially my self. And then the hangover begins.

My big-heartedness can block out other facts. With alcohol abuse, we speak of blackouts, times when the person drinking was up and doing things yet has no memory of those times. This is a warning sign of alcoholism. This is not good. Neither is it good when our being big-hearted has us blocking out important information that could help us make better decisions. If my love for you has me willing to risk life and limb unnecessarily, and I am not willing to look honestly at the data that suggest that danger or harm is possible, then I am out of my head.

My big-heartedness can block out other feelings. If my love for you has me willing to risk life and limb unnecessarily, and I am not willing to honestly and fully feel the other feelings I am likely to be experiencing as well, then I am putting us both in danger. What I offered generously and kindly at first has now become my obsession that refuses to allow me to connect with competing emotions that are likely mounting up in me and that, if acknowledged, will likely change my decisions and behaviors—changes I really do not want to consider because they may not produce the outcome my heart is set on.

My big-heartedness can block out my spirituality. If my love for you has me willing to risk life and limb unnecessarily, it is likely that I have disconnected from the will of my higher power and I am attached to my will. This is the trickiness about being good-spirited. Our loving spirits start out in good, kind places, with generosity and live-and-let-live attitudes toward all. We start out connected with our higher power and having trust in the other person having his or her higher power. Somewhere along the way, if we are not mindful, our loving and giving can shift into becoming some agenda of our own. This is where we likely move from genuinely and freely giving to having attachments to our giving. For me, these attachments reflect my disconnection from my spirituality. I become so focused on what I feel and want to do and accomplish through my deeds of goodness that I forget to even make contact with my higher power—a major source of my big-heartedness in the first place. Then I am out there trying to live *my* will, not *thy* will. At a certain point this does not work very well for me, or does not work for me at all.

When I am under the influence of my big-heartedness, I can make poor decisions. Though I am mindful not to overuse it, I do find this intoxication metaphor to be a useful way to understand how our loss of our self in our big-heartedness can disable us, as can the overuse of a substance. The last three lessons have established that our big-heartedness, in its more extreme, intoxicating forms, can block out competing facts, feelings, and spirit, so there is no way in the world that we are going to be able to make good decisions. Good decisions are based on our ability to gather, sort, review, assess, and select all types of information. When I am limiting what data I am willing to look at, then I am making important decisions based on incomplete and inaccurate information. No wonder I am then starting to put my self and others in harm's way.

What good is my love if we all die from it? I realize this sounds extreme. Most of the time we don't kill people with our love. But as I wrote the tales in this chapter, I realized how far I can get lost in what my heart may be directing. And as I have been watching Daisy now in her advanced years, I am learning that her basic nature of energy, loyalty, and spirit can kill her. Remember her airborne acrobatics? Recently I was talking to another border collie owner, and she acknowledged how their old border collies had still tried to run and jump and carry on just as they had when they were young. Their doing this had caused them health problems in their old age. My basic nature that includes being big-hearted can kill me as well if I am not mindful. I don't want Daisy or me or anyone to die from our love irrationally expressed. I don't want Daisy or me or anyone to be harmed in any way by the ways we express and act on our big-heartedness. All is lost when this happens: love can no longer be seen or experienced. How ironic. How true.

I want to listen not only to my heart but also to my thoughts, other feelings, body, and spirit. Though the messages from my heart may be very strong and very delicious, I must remember to actively be in contact with these other, equally important parts of my self.

If I cannot hear them, I need to quiet my self intentionally and pay attention without judgment. I need to just notice my thoughts, my other feelings, my body sensations, and my higher power contact. As I gather all of this information and process it, I may then be better able to balance the power of my heart with the other realities of my situation. Because you see, I have learned and deeply believe that:

Kindness of heart + presence of mind can go a long way toward excellence in health. This excellence in health is what my work is all about. It is about both physical health and mental health. It is about attending to self as we attend to others. It is about giving to self as we give to others. It is about loving my self as I love others. The balancing of all of this is what can bring me long-lasting love, serenity, and health. Moment by moment, I want to remember this and live this.

*T**he border collie is a working dog who thrives*
on having a job to do and a purpose in life[1]
—*Mary Burch*

never-endings

And On We Go

I was about to come in from my early-morning walk with Daisy and Eddie and go to my writing for the one precious hour I can find for it several days per week. It was a Monday morning and around twenty-five degrees outside. In two weeks it would be Christmas. I had our clear candles lit in our windows and multicolored lights around our front door with a beautiful, fresh Christmas wreath just brought back from the farmer's market the past weekend. No one else can see our house except the engineers of the trains that pass several times per day, but I see our charming little cottage and I love it every time I see it, especially looking so cute and seasonal with the lights on and the smoke coming out of our chimney.

I was about to prepare to write this last chapter. I wasn't going to *write*. I was just going to organize my self and my thoughts on this last message. What I already knew was that I was going to tell you that happily, Daisy and I have both made it to the conclusion of the writing of this book. After ten years, Daisy and I are both here to keep telling our stories. And to punctuate this alive-and-kicking status of each of us, here's what Daisy offered as we entered our front yard from our walk.

I had let Daisy and Eddie off of their leashes as we got closer to the house. They had run ahead to explore in their usual ways. As I got closer to them, I saw Daisy standing beside my car as she usually does, looking back to make sure I was coming. All of a sudden she took off like she was in a competitive agility trial. She lowered her body into her sleek running posture and ran around my car twice like a barrel-racing horse, cutting her corners closely but accurately and beautifully. She then continued running around parts of our yard close to the house, which are hilly. She made a loop around the big tree, running in our lower driveway and circling up to the upper driveway. She did this twice, too. As she circled from the upper driveway back down to the lower driveway, she would leap to the lower levels. She ran one more time around my car and then ran toward the front porch, taking a big leap onto the porch from the terracing in front of it. What a display of border collie! What a display of health and vigor and aliveness! Did she know I was coming to write this last section, and had she another burst to contribute?

The whole time Daisy was bringing me this wonderful morning celebration, I had a couple of thoughts. First, I was thinking about how smart she is and how able she is. She has created her own agility courses here at our home, and she can really show off when the spirit moves her. Second, I was thinking I shouldn't cheer her on in her running as I have over the years. I was smiling and clearly loving her energy and spirit, but I was also aware of all I have told you about Daisy being sixteen. I know she is old. I don't know if she knows or remembers she is old in such moments. So I don't want to be in the same denial that she may be in and encourage her in ways that could hurt her.

Yes, Daisy and I have aged in noticeable ways over the ten years of the creation of this book. We are both considerably grayer. Daisy has grayed especially around her face, with salt-and-pepper coloring around her eyes and down her nose. I am even grayer. Having kept my long hair and never colored it, there is no way around the fact that I have gray/silver hair. For the most part I am okay with this. I am even stopped on occasion by strangers who tell me how pretty my hair is. But still, when I look in the mirror and see my gray or when I see a photograph of my self now, I am struck by the reality of my aging.

Neither Daisy nor I live as though we are our chronological ages. Just this past summer at Lake Eaton in the Adirondacks of New York, Monty and I and Daisy and Eddie were off on our morning walk to a small, secluded beach on the lake. When we got to the beach, another family was already set up there, but we stopped and talked with them a while. Daisy became a topic of our conversation. When we told them her age, one of the men said, "She's not dragging anchor!" She sure wasn't. She was prancing into the water up to her chest, throwing the water up in the air with her snout, and pulling on her leash to be able to walk along the water's edge to an even more secluded rock beach that she remembered from our other years there. Daisy's not dragging anchor.

And I am not, either. Daisy and I both are spirited dancers: Daisy in all the ways I have described through this book, and me through decades of dance classes and performances, through classes taken and taught, through pieces danced and/or choreographed. I have been known to say, "Daisy and I both dance." During a visit here with us, Ava said, "Daisy did a big old dance in the middle of the living room." Daisy's dancing technique varies from the cute bounce in her step to her teeter-tottering in the living room to her ability to do a complete *tour en l'air,* which means she can jump up in the air and do a full turn before she lands back where she started.

Daisy and I still think we can do our leaps and turns. Sometimes we can, and sometimes we can't now. We each have developed some stiffness and weaker spots in our bodies. Daisy has arthritis in her back legs. My left knee has something wrong with it that limits some dance moves. We each want to deny these changes, but really we can't afford to do that. As has been a theme in this book, our recognizing the realities of our very self is imperative to our maintaining our physical and emotional health. So more and more, I am helping Daisy and me to attend to these physical realities to foster our health and long life.

Daisy and I are also working to maintain our spiritual health. Daisy continues to convey joy and good energy. Her spirit seems energized. She has, indeed, had a fine life, and I choose to believe that she appreciates that. She has traveled widely with us on our car trips from Maine to Florida, from Virginia to California. Daisy has a little red towel that I put on her seat in the car when she is going with us. When she sees me putting that red towel in place, she can hardly wait until she can jump up onto her seat and go. Daisy is always ready to go! Her spirit is strong and good.

Daisy's spirit feeds my spirit. She is not my only spiritual source by any means, but she is an important source. I can't help but come to the present moment when I see her. Then I smile and let go of whatever thoughts or feelings had me captive, and I join Daisy for love and good spirit.

I want you to know all of this about Daisy and me as I am finishing this book, because you have come to know us through our Tales and Lessons. Having you know how we are aging and how we are handling that reality as we work on all of these lessons seems important to me. And though I know that the reality is that one day our lives will be over here, I chose to entitle this final chapter "Never-Endings." The title is not to deny that Daisy and I both will have endings to our lives. We will. For now, though, I choose to speak about the never-endings of my work on my self as long as I am here and able. The Tales and Lessons I have offered are rich and informative, and, like a good parable, they can be and must be used over and over again to teach me and help me grow. I see my growth as an exciting, never-ending process with clear and important aspects to it.

Keeping Our Spirits Alive and Always Working on Our Training

This is a never-ending process of self-discovery and growth.
I have come to know and to accept this. I have come to be excited about this. My experience with learning about my self and seeing changes I want to make for my self is that this is not a "check that off the list/I've done that" process. It *is* in fact a process, an active, ongoing process that has me making good progress and yet seeing another something that I can change for my self that will help me to have greater serenity and healthier relationships. I have learned that there are fundamental ways about me that can help or hurt me and that it is only through my self-education and mindful presence that I am able to manage and change those ways. And for me, this is a never-ending process that has me learning and growing most of the time.

My progress can be two steps forward and one step back.
I have learned this expression through my twelve-step fellowship. Not only does this process of discovery and growth provide ongoing opportunities for forward movement for me; sometimes that forward movement is made possible by my moving backward for a bit. Sometimes I fail to live in my growth. Sometimes the tangled, codependent me is in action, and I remember her and how I feel when I am acting in this way. Note the word *acting*. Remember, in this book I have been talking about codependent behaviors rather than the concept of codependency so that we can learn practical ways to work with our self. In this case, when I notice that I have taken one step backward, it is likely that I am noticing that I am being too devoted, too reactive, or too tenacious. Actually, I could be behaving in ways that reflect too much of any of the twelve qualities I have written about in this book. So I notice, regroup, and move forward again. I am so aware of the fact that I can move backward that when I am offering ideas to someone else about how to act less codependently, I qualify my comments by saying, "When I am

in good form . . ." I am not always in good form. I am working toward being in good form more and more of the time.

We want to embrace our natural tendencies and manage them so our strengths do not become our weaknesses. In this case of writing in the plural, I have Daisy and me in mind, though I am certainly speaking to all of us who are engaged in this process of growth and change. Daisy and I both thrive on having a job to do and a purpose in life, and we come equipped with many wonderful qualities that enable us to fulfill these personal goals and desires. We do our jobs well, and we are pleased by our accomplishments. We are blessed with energy, focus, and loyalty. But as we have learned through this book, these fantastic assets can go too far and cause trouble, whether the being is a canine or a human. We can run our self to death, lose track of other important responsibilities and/or people, and stop noticing and attending to our self. So, knowing these possibilities for my strengths to weaken me:

I pay attention to where I am on the continuum of a specific behavior and adjust my self on that continuum as I would adjust a thermostat. This is an important part of my training. Daisy has her own training, which she continues to need, and I certainly have my own. Using the continuum as a tool to help me notice and gauge my self is very useful. Codependency is not a black-and-white issue. We are not simply codependent or not. There are important gradations to the behaviors that can ultimately have us acting in codependent ways. Further, codependency itself is fostered by black-and-white/all-or-nothing thinking, which has us unable to live in the gray. All of this is to say that I choose to use the continuum to help me notice the point at which my serving is becoming too much, my devotion has me accepting the unacceptable, my tenacity has me wearing out, or my big-heartedness has me with diminishing funds. If I am in a room that is too hot, I naturally go and turn down the heat. If I am losing my healthy connection with my self as I am in relationships with others, I want to go turn down the heat of my codependent behaviors.

I want to always be open and willing to learn the new lessons that are there for me. New lessons are here for me all of the time. I like the word *lesson*. I think it is a pretty and solid word that makes me smile. How nice to be able to learn something new. How nice to do things differently. How nice to be able to feel better about my self and to enjoy my life. When those opportunities for growth and new lessons show up, I am not always able to immediately welcome them in. I may even be defensive and resistant. Yet through my recovery I have learned to soften my defensiveness, quiet my self, and let this new information in so that I can study it and decide how I might want to use it to improve my self and live in and with greater serenity. Lessons Learned. Lessons Loved.

One More Tale

As I have been nearing the end of this book, I have been given another tale to tell you. It is about blurring the boundaries between Daisy and me. Losing our self in our codependent behaviors is about blurring the boundaries between you and me. As I lose my self more and more in you, I disappear from me. I then feel and speak and act for you and not for me. At times I can't even tell which of us I am referring to or talking about with my boundaries so lost in yours.

This blurring of boundaries began showing up in me in a distinct way as I was moving into the last parts of writing this book. I started "blurring the endings." In my happy anxiety about finally almost completing this book after ten years, I started to feel uneasy about whether Daisy's life would end as I was finishing the book. After all, Daisy has aged considerably over these years, as have I. I have not lost my self in this fear, but there have been times when I could have allowed my self to really get into worrying about whether I could finish it before she dies and/or whether she would die when our work here is done. Someone even asked me, "Are you worried that Daisy will just keel over and die when you write the last word?" I had not been talking about this fear. My friend just posed this same question out of her own wonderings. But as I have said, I have not lost my self in this fear. I have noticed it and been able to set it aside over and over again so that I could write freely and with great pleasure.

Just in the last month, one more tale from the Johnston home offered itself. It is called "The Story of the Steps."

Daisy has arthritis in her back legs. This has been developing for a year or so, but it has not been an obvious problem until the last several months. Daisy does fine on relatively flat surfaces and surfaces that are not slippery. In fact, for the most part, she still does fine in her running and jumping and prancing on most surfaces, except on our wooden stairs that go up to our bedroom and to her foam mattress.

I know I wrote about these stairs in earlier stories. The stairs are in our front hallway. This is not a grand stairway. This is a cottage-size stairway that goes up and turns right at the top with another two stairs into our bedroom. The stairs have always been bare wood. I think they are pretty and I have enjoyed the natural wood. These are the stairs Daisy has loved to lie on as one of her central posts for herding us, for knowing where we all are in the house.

This fall I noticed Daisy having more trouble with the stairs. She could go up okay, but coming down she started to show some difficulties. She would cautiously take it step by step, letting her front legs take the lead and then carefully figuring out how to let her back legs jump and land on the next step down. I noticed that those back legs were starting to slide out from under her some. One morning as we came downstairs to start our day, she actually slid down several steps, keeping her standing posture but lowering her self so that it appeared that her rib cage actually traveled along the edges of the steps. I was standing behind her, watching this helplessly.

I stood totally quiet, wanting so badly to help her and knowing there was no way to do so. In the pause, I watched Daisy problem solve in her border collie way. I knew her brain was working to figure out how to get her self out of this situation. And she did. After a few moments, Daisy organized herself and miraculously was able to "pull herself together" and proceed down the stairs in her usual way, unharmed.

It was clearly time to do something to fix this situation! The border collie in me wanted to fix this right away, but the time constraints of my week did not make that possible. I was in the middle of my busy clinical work, with no extra time for shopping and/or home improvements with our dog in mind. But I fit in action on this problem as I could, shopping online for stair treads, running to stores at the end of the day to check on carpeting, and talking with Monty every chance I got to figure out what we could do.

By the end of that week, I had brought home a package of four carpeted stair treads for us to try—not fancy, but very practical. On Friday night, Monty and I put down the treads on the top four steps. We measured, trimmed, and stapled them down over the pretty wood. Only Lola the cat noticed our work. She's an excellent supervisor of many things, and she was quite attentive. When it was bedtime, I watched Daisy go up the stairs. When she got to the top four steps, she noticed the treads, paused, and tried to walk around them as best as she could as she made her way up the rest of the way. I wondered if these treads were going to be weird to her like the mailbox was to Mary Burch's Laddie.

Nevertheless, Monty and I assessed that these treads were a good idea and would work. So the next day I went and bought two more packages of treads so we could do the entire stairway.

I arrived home late in the afternoon with the treads, and we went right to work on them. We knew what we were doing, since we had practiced with the first four treads. We started putting these next treads on where we left off, working our way down the stairs with our installations. This time Daisy noticed what we were doing. She came into the hallway from the living room and watched with her alertness and presence. Lola and Zoe were both with us as well, Lola supervising again and Zoe quietly sitting on the new treads.

All of a sudden it was like Daisy understood what we were doing. She came to the bottom of the steps and started walking up the stairs through our menagerie of people and cats and scissors and staplers. When she got to the top of the stairs she turned around and pranced back down, enjoying the traction of the carpet. She then turned around at the bottom of the steps and repeated this entire pattern, even walking through my legs as she made her way on this special trek. She ran up the stairs and happily, happily came back down with confidence and security three times. We were all happily, happily enjoying this wonderful time. Monty said Daisy was "marveling" at what had now become possible for her again. It was, as he said, "a fine time."

It was dusk as we finished putting the treads down. It was time to take the dogs out for a walk. We were feeling the tremendous success of our work and were talking about it as we walked.

I said, "I'll bet Daisy sleeps better tonight."

I continued, with some self-awareness, "Maybe it's me who will sleep better tonight."

And I continued on with my self-reflections, my never-ending lessons. "It's a fine line."

"Between you and Daisy?" asked Monty.

"Yep," I said.

And it's an important line: Daisy being Daisy and me being me.

beginnings

1. Mary Burch, *The Border Collie: An Owner's Guide to a Happy Healthy Pet*. New York: Howell Book House, 1996, p. 26.

2. Robin Norwood, *Women Who Love Too Much: When You Keep Hoping He'll Change*. New York: Pocket Books, 1985, p. 48.

3. Melody Beattie, *Codependent No More*. Center City, MN: Hazelden, 1987, p. 31.

4. American Psychiatric Association, *Diagnostic and Statistical Manual of Mental Health Disorders (DSM-IV)*, Fourth Edition. Arlington, VA: American Psychiatric Publishing, 2000.

5. Norwood, *Women Who Love Too Much*.

6. Beattie, *Codependent No More*, p. 31.

7. Sharon Wegscheider-Cruse, *Another Chance: Hope and Health for the Alcoholic Family*. Deerfield Beach, FL: Health Communications, Inc., 1989.

8. Janet Geringer Woititz, *Adult Children of Alcoholics, Expanded Edition*. Deerfield Beach, FL: Health Communications, Inc., 1990.

9. Timmen L. Cermak, *Diagnosing and Treating Co-Dependence*. Minneapolis: Johnson Institute Books, 1986, p. 11.

10. Nancy L. Johnston, *Diagnosing Codependence*. Unpublished manuscript, 1990.

11. Toby Rice Drews, *Getting Them Sober, Volume 4: Separations and Healings*. Baltimore: Recovery Communications, Inc., 1992.

12. Nancy L. Johnston, *Disentangle: When You've Lost Your Self in Someone Else*. Las Vegas: Central Recovery Press, 2011.

13. Jon Kabat-Zinn, *Full Catastrophe Living*. New York: Delacorte Press, 1990.

14. Elizabeth Zelvin, "Treating the Partners of Substance Abusers," in *Clinical Work with Substance-Abusing Clients*, ed. Shulamith Lala Ashenberg Straussner. New York: Guilford Press, 2005, p. 264.

15. Ibid., p. 282.

16. Janice Haaken, "From Al-Anon to ACOA: Codependence and the Resconstruction of Caregiving," *Signs,* volume 18, issue 2 (1993): pp. 321–45.

17. Zelvin, "Treating the Partners of Substance Abusers," p. 267.

18. Ibid., p. 282.

19. Greg E. Dear et al., "Defining Codependency: A Thematic Analysis of Published Definitions," *Advances in Psychology Research*, volume 34 (2005), pp. 189–205.

20. Greg E. Dear and Clare M. Roberts, "Validation of the Holyoake Codependency Index," *The Journal of Psychology,* volume 139, issue 4 (2005), p. 294.

21. Barbara Yoder, *The Recovery Resource Book*. New York: Simon & Schuster, 1990, p. 217.

22. Teri A. Loughead, "Addictions as a Process: Commonalities or Codependence," *Contemporary Family Therapy*, volume 13, issue 5 (1991), pp. 455–70.

23. Layne A. Prest and Howard Protinsky, "Family Systems Theory: A Unifying Framework for Codependence," *The American Journal of Family Therapy*, volume 21, issue 4 (1993), pp. 352–60.

24. Robert Subby and John Friel, "Co-dependency," in *Co-dependency: A Book of Readings Reprinted from FOCUS on Family and Chemical Dependency*. Deerfield Beach, FL: Health Communications, Inc., 1984, p. 34.

25. Loughead, "Addictions as a Process," pp. 455–70.

26. Wegscheider-Cruse, *Another Chance*.

27. Haaken, "From Al-Anon to ACOA," pp. 321–45.

28. Anne Wilson Schaef, *Co-Dependence Misunderstood-Mistreated*. San Francisco: HarperOne, 1992, p. 21.

29. Ibid., pp. 41–2.

tales and lessons

1. Mary Burch, *The Border Collie: An Owner's Guide to a Happy Healthy Pet*. New York: Howell Book House, 1996, p. 26.

2. Ibid., p. 27.

3. Ibid., p. 5.

4. Ibid., p. 25.

5. Ibid, p. 25.

6. Ibid., p. 27.

7. Ibid.

8. Greg E. Dear et al., "Defining Codependency: A Thematic Analysis of Published Definitions," *Advances in Psychology Research*, volume 34 (2005), pp. 189–205.

9. Greg E. Dear and Clare M. Roberts, "Validation of the Holyoake Codependency Index," *The Journal of Psychology*, volume 139, issue 4 (2005), p. 294.

10. Gary L. Fisher and Thomas C. Harrison, *Substance Abuse: Information for School Counselors, Social Workers, Therapists, and Counselors*. Boston: Allyn and Bacon, 1997.

11. Elizabeth Zelvin, "Treating the Partners of Substance Abusers," in *Clinical Work with Substance-Abusing Clients*, ed. Shulamith Lala Ashenberg Straussner. New York: Guilford Press, 2005, p. 270.

12. Barbara Yoder, *The Recovery Resource Book*. New York: Simon & Schuster, 1990, p. 218.

13. Virginia Morell, "Minds of Their Own: Animals Are Smarter Than You Think," *National Geographic*, volume 213, issue 3 (2008), pp. 36–61.

14. Burch, p. 13.

15. Ibid., p. 25.

16. Dear et al., pp. 189–205.

17. Jon Kabat-Zinn, *Full Catastrophe Living*. New York: Delacorte Press, 1990.

18. Burch, p. 33.

19. Ibid., p. 34.

20. Ibid., p. 6.

21. Ibid., p. 30.

22. Ibid., p. 33.

23. Ibid., p. 28.

24. Ibid., p. 27.

25. Ibid., pp. 9 – 11.

26. Ibid., p. 28.

27. Dear et al., pp. 189–205.

28. Burch, p. 6.

29. Ibid., p. 29.

30. Ibid., p. 30.

31. Ibid.

32. Nancy L. Johnston, *Disentangle: When You've Lost Your Self in Someone Else*. Las Vegas: Central Recovery Press, 2011.

33. Ibid.

34. Dear et al., p. 198.

35. Ibid., p. 199.

36. Burch, p. 10.

37. Dear and Roberts, p. 200.

38. Burch, p. 29.

39. Ibid., p. 9.

40. Ibid., p. 24.

41. American Psychiatric Association, *Diagnostic and Statistical Manual of Mental Health Disorders (DSM-IV)*, Fourth Edition. Arlington, VA: American Psychiatric Publishing, 2000.

42. Burch, p. 25.

43. Ibid., p. 6.

44. Ibid., p. 29.

45. Ibid.

46. Ibid., p. 9-10.

47. Ibid., p. 34.

48. Dear et al., pp. 189–205.

49. Dear and Roberts, p. 294.

never-endings

1. Burch, p. 25.

Relationships and Self-Help

Disentangle: When You've Lost Your Self in Someone Else
Nancy L. Johnston, MS, LPC, LSATP • $15.95 US
ISBN-13: 978-1-936290-03-1

Dancing in the Dark: How to Take Care of Yourself When Someone You Love Is Depressed
Bernadette Stankard and Amy Viets • $15.95 US
ISBN-13: 978-1-936290-70-3

A Spiritual Path to a Healthy Relationship: A Practical Approach
Steve McCord, MFT and Angie McCord, CC • $15.95 US
ISBN-13: 978-1-936290-65-9

Picking Up the Pieces without Picking Up:
A Guidebook through Victimization for People in Recovery
Jennifer Storm • $15.95 US • ISBN-13: 978-1-936290-64-2

From Heartbreak to Heart's Desire:
Developing a Healthy GPS (Guy Picking System)
Dawn Maslar, MS • $14.95 US • ISBN-13: 978-0-9818482-6-6

Addiction and Recovery

When the Servant Becomes the Master: A Comprehensive Addiction Guide for Those Who Suffer from the Disease, the Loved Ones Affected By It, and the Professionals Who Assist Them
Jason Z W Powers, MD • $18.95 US • ISBN-13: 978-1-936290-81-9

Finding a Purpose in the Pain:
A Doctor's Approach to Addiction Recovery and Healing
James L. Fenley, Jr., MD • $15.95 US • ISBN-13: 978-1-936290-71-0

Yoga and the Twelve-Step Path
Kyczy Hawk • $15.95 US • ISBN-13: 978-1-936290-80-2

Recovery A to Z: A Handbook of Twelve-Step Key Terms and Phrases
The Editors of Central Recovery Press • $15.95 US
ISBN-13: 978-1-936290-04-8

Inspirational

The Truth Begins with You: Reflections to Heal Your Spirit
Claudia Black, PhD • $17.95 US • ISBN-13: 978-1-936290-61-1

Above and Beyond:
365 Meditations for Transcending Chronic Pain and Illness
J.S. Dorian • $15.95 US • ISBN-13: 978-1-936290-66-6

Guide Me in My Recovery: Prayers for Times of Joy and Times of Trial
Rev. John T. Farrell, PhD • $12.95 US • ISBN-13: 978-1-936290-00-0
Special hardcover gift edition: $19.95 US • ISBN-13: 978-1-936290-02-4

The Soul Workout: Getting and Staying Spiritually Fit
Helen H. Moore • $12.95 US • ISBN-13: 978-0-9799869-8-7

Tails of Recovery: Addicts and the Pets That Love Them
Nancy A. Schenck • $19.95 US • ISBN-13: 978-0-9799869-6-3

Of Character: Building Assets in Recovery
Denise D. Crosson, PhD • $12.95 US • ISBN-13: 978-0-9799869-2-5

Memoirs

From Bagels to Buddha: How I Found My Soul and Lost My Fat
Judi Hollis, PhD • $16.95 US • ISBN-13: 978-1-936290-81-9

Fear: Feel It, Face It, and Grow
Mark Edick • $17.95 US • ISBN-13: 978-1-936290-72-7

Leave the Light On: A Memoir of Recovery and Self-Discovery
Jennifer Storm • $14.95 US • ISBN-13: 978-0-9818482-2-8

The Mindful Addict: A Memoir of the Awakening of a Spirit
Tom Catton • $18.95 US • ISBN-13: 978-0-9818482-7-3

Becoming Normal: An Ever-Changing Perspective
Mark Edick • $14.95 US • ISBN-13: 978-0-9818482-1-1

Dopefiend: A Father's Journey from Addiction to Redemption
Tim Elhajj • 16.95 US • ISBN-13: 978-1-936290-63-5